LOVING THE
G-SPOT

LOVING THE
G-SPOT

THE DEFINITIVE GUIDE ON
THE SECRET CENTER OF
FEMININE PLEASURE

MARCIA DURANTE

TRANSLATED BY

ELIZABETH WATSON

Skyhorse Publishing

Original title: SOLA O EN PAREJA, DESCUBRE Y DISFRUTA DE TU PUNTO G
© 2005 Marcia Durante
© 2008 by Editorial Océano, S.L. (Barcelona, Spain)
Illustrations: Xavier Bou

English translation © 2015 by Skyhorse Publishing

Skyhorse Publishing books may be purchased in bulk at special discounts for sales promotion, corporate gifts, fund-raising, or educational purposes. Special editions can also be created to specifications. For details, contact the Special Sales Department, Skyhorse Publishing, 307 West 36th Street, 11th Floor, New York, NY 10018 or info@skyhorsepublishing.com.

Skyhorse® and Skyhorse Publishing® are registered trademarks of Skyhorse Publishing, Inc.®, a Delaware corporation.

Visit our website at www.skyhorsepublishing.com.

10 9 8 7 6 5

Library of Congress Cataloging-in-Publication Data
Durante, Marcia.
  [Sola o en pareja, descubre y disfruta de tu punto G. English]
  Loving the G-spot : the definitive guide on the secret center of feminine pleasure /
Marcia Durante ; translated by Elizabeth Watson
      pages cm
   Summary: "As much for those in a relationship as well as those who want to enjoy their own bodies, this manual teaches you to locate the G-spot and to stimulate it to unleash a true "Big Bang" of pleasure. It includes detailed illustrations that show, step-by-step, the path to female ecstasy"-- Provided by publisher.
  ISBN 978-1-63220-325-0 (paperback) -- ISBN 978-1-63220-858-3 (ebook) 1. Sex instruction for women. 2. G spot. 3. Female orgasm. I. Title.
  HQ46.D8713 2015
  306.7082--dc23
                                    2015003880

Cover design by David Sankey
Cover photo credit: Thinkstock

ISBN: 978-1-63220-325-0
Ebook ISBN 978-1-63220-858-3

Printed in the United States of America

Contents

The existence of the G-spot, a highly erogenous zone in women, is undeniable, although few books talk about it thoroughly or explain the best positions we can practice (alone or with a partner) to get maximum enjoyment from its stimulation and how to strengthen the muscles of this area to reach greater pleasure. When you directly stimulate the G-spot, it begins to swell until it triggers a vaginal orgasm, which is physiologically and psychologically different from a clitoral orgasm, and is nearly always accompanied by ejaculation.

Reading this book will give you the tools necessary to find and enjoy this secret part of your body, since it gives detailed explanations about the subtleties of some of the sexual practices that help you achieve full satisfaction, as well as all things related to female ejaculation. As you advance you will also reach a new type of spiritual, physical, and mental liberation and you will discover that your body can become a source of pleasure that surpasses imagination, through which you will achieve the strongest, wildest, and longest orgasms.

Although at first it may seem to be, this book is not just for a female audience. It is a book designed for men as well, because pleasure is for both sexes… and to share.

In this book you will find:

- Techniques to find and stimulate the female and male G-spot.
- Techniques to teach you how to ejaculate.
- The role of the partner in female ejaculation.

- The most erogenous parts of your body.
- The most pleasurable massages.
- The secrets of reaching orgasm.
- The most satisfying positions of our *Kamasutra*.

Learn everything you ever wanted to know about pleasure and never dared to ask! You will discover the deepest secrets of your body and the most varied sensations... Happy reading and even better practicing!

Marcia Durante

Introduction

For ages women's sexuality has been relegated to the mere reproductive role, and in some cases even women themselves have become unconcerned, focusing their relations on men's satisfaction. In recent years, however, women are insisting more and more on our right to enjoy—either alone or accompanied—the pleasures of knowing and stimulating every corner of our bodies. Because the truth is that the female sexual universe is so broad and complex it exceeds the man's, and experimenting with caress and stimulation of our erogenous zones—of our pleasure spots—can give us previously undiscovered satisfaction. Plus, it means that we can achieve a passionate experience when having sex with our partner.

It is important and beneficial to start by getting rid of false taboos about sex and approaching it with an open mind, willing to test all the new discoveries that we desire. Among all taboos surrounding our sex, one of the most generalized is the denial of the G-spot's existence, an area that, the most qualified sexologists say, is scientifically proven. And along with this denial is the failure to mention women's ability to ejaculate, as well as their ability to enjoy multiple orgasms. However, none of the previous statements are true: we have a G-spot located in the interior of our vagina, and we can ejaculate and enjoy the ability to have not only one orgasm but many. You just have to understand the resources that your own body offers in order to fully enjoy it.

After reading these pages, where you will find explicit and simple illustrations on both sexual organs and different postures, you will not only have learned to locate your G-spot, but also all the tricks for maximum enjoyment of your body—which leads into the even more unknown world of female ejaculation.

Would you like to try it out? Do you want to get lost in the winding paths of pleasure? You just have to keep on reading!

Test: What do you know about the female orgasm?

"Orgasm" is one of the most oft repeated words in this book. Surely it's not unknown to you and you have enjoyed it during your sexual experiences. But what is an orgasm exactly? How is it reached? How many could you have?

Reaching arousal and orgasm afterward is a complex process that involves the mind and the body. The human mind receives sexual stimuli, processes them, and, based on its experiences, causes the body to respond. The brain could begin the process of sexual arousal in response to thoughts (sexual fantasy), to visual stimuli (looking at the partner naked), to audible stimulus (hearing the partner's voice), to olfactory stimuli (partner's smell), to taste (taste of the partner's body), or to any combination of these. This means that almost anything can lead us to the orgasm if we are predisposed. Mind and body have the ability to experience an orgasm separately. Therefore, in order to reach an orgasm, mind and body need to work together.

Before you keep on reading and answer this test's questions, it's important that you be true to yourself and let go of prejudices.

Take your time and don't worry if in any case you don't know what
to answer, or if at some point you think that the answer can be true
and false at the same time; when you are finished reading the book
you will be more conscious of your abilities to reach the greatest
pleasure, and about how and why you experience an orgasm. If you
prefer you can answer these questions after you are done reading
the book.

- **Question 1.** An orgasm is the response to total sexual satisfaction that you feel in your entire body.
  TRUE   FALSE

- **Question 2.** Women enjoy coitus as much as men do.
  TRUE   FALSE

- **Question 3.** The majority of women have an orgasm during the sexual act.
  TRUE   FALSE

- **Question 4.** Women only have clitoral orgasms.
  TRUE   FALSE

- **Question 5.** Women can reach orgasm by masturbating only.
  TRUE   FALSE

- **Question 6.** An orgasm is conditioned not only physically but also mentally.
  TRUE   FALSE

- **Question 7.** The goal of coitus is to always have an orgasm.
  TRUE   FALSE

- **Question 8.** Depending on the conditioning of pelvic muscles, women can have different kinds of orgasms.
  TRUE   FALSE

ANSWERS

- **Question 1.** A woman's body is equipped to feel pleasure completely; don't forget that the skin is the main source of sensations. Although many women need the stimulus to begin on particular parts of their body (not necessarily the genitals), eventually their entire body responds.
  Correct answer: TRUE

- **Question 2.** Here the explanation is really short: yes, as long as they give us the opportunity, of course.
  Correct answer: TRUE

- **Question 3.** Lack of information about female sexuality has led to the fact that many women have taken a long time to realize that they can also enjoy orgasm and that the sexual act does not end with men's ejaculation. In order to have satisfactory sexual relationships for both partners, communication at all times is paramount.
  Correct answer: FALSE

- **Question 4.** Here both answers can be valid, because it's up to each woman. The female orgasm has always been associated with stimulation of the clitoris; however, women can have orgasms skipping its stimulation, and have vaginal orgasms as a result of G-spot stimulation.
  correct answer: TRUE AND FALSE

- **Question 5.** Masturbation has long been a condemned practice, for both men and women. However, who else do you expect to know the corners of your body that give you the most pleasure and what better than reaching orgasm by yourself? So, enjoy as much as you want with masturbation; not only is it harmless, but it's also immensely pleasurable.
  Correct answer: TRUE

- **Question 6.** Depending on each woman, the mental component will be more or less important to reaching orgasm. Although it's necessary to demystify the fact that women only enjoy sex thoroughly when there is love in the relationship, what is true is that for us, women, the emotional component determines more our sexual practices.
  Correct answer: TRUE AND FALSE

- **Question 7.** Although it's always pleasurable to end the sexual act with an orgasm, we should not get obsessed with the idea, because we can have very satisfying relations with all different kinds of sensations.
  Correct answer: TRUE

- **Question 8.** Here science imposes itself, and every study confirms that if you control your PC muscles (or muscles of love) you can reach more intense orgasms and, even, many of them (the multiorgasmic ability of women is real). In order to strengthen them you can just read the part in which we show you the exercises that will help you enhance them.
  Correct answer: TRUE

Test: What do you know about the G-spot?

Before we get into the pleasurable world of the G-spot and female ejaculation, find a calm place at home and carefully read the following test questions.

Until very recently, a lot of people asserted that the G-spot was only a myth, and currently some still believe so. However, when you are finished with this book you will confirm (and experience) that it's not true. For now, there is this questionnaire so you can rate your knowledge of the G-spot. Don't worry if you skip a question, or if you realize that an answer is wrong. When you are done reading this book I recommend you review your responses again and you will realize you can answer them without hesitation. If you prefer, you can skip this test right now and get back to it when you are done with the book.

- **Question 1.** There is a sensitive part of the vagina called the "G-spot" due to its similarity to the man's glans. In fact, a woman's G-spot and a man's glans are a source of equivalent voluptuous sensations.
  TRUE   FALSE

- **Question 2.** During sexual arousal the G-spot increases in size and becomes easily noticeable.
TRUE   FALSE

- **Question 3.** The G-spot is located deep in the vagina.
TRUE   FALSE

- **Question 4.** Certain positions during coitus benefit G-spot stimulation.
TRUE   FALSE

- **Question 5.** G-spot stimulation provokes an initial sensation of having to urinate and the woman discharges some liquid.
TRUE   FALSE

- **Question 6.** G-spot stimulation always provokes an orgasm.
TRUE   FALSE

- **Question 7.** The G-spot is an anatomic formation that is related to female ejaculation.
TRUE   FALSE

- **Question 8.** Every woman has a G-spot.
TRUE   FALSE

- **Question 9.** Every man has a G-spot.
TRUE   FALSE

ANSWERS

- **Question 1.** In 1950 Ernest Gräfenberg published an article describing a previously ignored zone of the vagina. Later, in the 1980s, some American researchers who were working on female sexuality became aware of this zone and picked up his studies again. It is in these studies that they called it: "Gräfenberg's spot," which it just abbreviated as "G-spot." Correct answer: FALSE

- **Question 2.** In various scientific studies, sexologists who specialize in female sexuality have found a quarter-sized zone that swells when it receives tactile stimulation—causing a very gratifying sensation—and that is directly related to the orgasm.
  Correct answer: TRUE

- **Question 3.** Although it is not always in the same place, the G-spot is generally located in the anterior wall of the vagina, a few centimeters from the entrance, by the sphincter and the urethral sponge.
  Correct answer: FALSE

- **Question 4.** Basically, when a woman kneels on top of the man or when he positions himself behind her, vaginal sensations are often much more intense than in some other positions. If you feel like "sharing" your G-spot with your partner, there is an explanation of the most stimulating sex positions later on.
  Correct answer: TRUE

- **Question 5.** Many women explain that, after stimulation of their G-spot, they suddenly feel like urinating. If you are in this situation, my advice is that you take a break for a few minutes and then continue with the stimulation. Soon you will realize that what takes over your body is a great sensation of pleasure and that the discharge running down your legs is not urine, but ejaculation.
  Correct answer: TRUE

- **Question 6.** Stimulation of the G-spot is just one component to reaching orgasm; nevertheless, it is normal when you need to reach different levels of sexual arousal.
  Correct answer: FALSE

- **Question 7.** Ernest Gräfenberg indicated that the stimulation of such zone is directly correlated with expulsion of a liquid through the urethra and established that this was female ejaculation.
Correct answer: TRUE

- **Question 8.** It is likely that, just as we are born with legs and arms, all women have this anatomic feature. In fact, according to surveys, only a small percentage of women claim to not have special sensations while stimulating this zone and perhaps the reason is that they are unable to find it. Is some education necessary, then, to reach this kind of pleasure? Yes, I recommend it, and in order to do so I will teach you to locate and correctly simulate it.
Correct answer: TRUE

- **Question 9.** Although "G-spot" is not the most proper term to designate that sensitive part of men—which also leads to orgasm—it is true that they bear certain similarity. The analogous masculine zone to the female G-spot is the one surrounding the urethra and the urethral sphincter. If a man receives adequate stimulation in that spot, he will have very intense voluptuous sensations, similar to the ones women feel by stimulation of their G-spot. To achieve it, the perineum below the testicles should be massaged, just in front of the anus; you can also insert a finger in the anus to massage the prostate directly.
Correct answer: TRUE

Toward the orgasm

It is difficult to talk about orgasm because it refers to such a personal experience, a sensation so unique and incomparable, that any given definition could be inappropriate. In fact, the first advice that I can give you is to not obsess over it and the second, that you begin to love and get to know yourself—by touching yourself, looking at yourself, and enjoying your own stimulation (it is an excellent exercise for couples too), until you get carried away. This is the only way to enjoy complete sexuality. And it is important that you do all this voluntarily, without any kind of imposition.

Sexual activity should be a pleasurable experience and should not be an activity requiring a concrete result. The joy and exploration of your body and your partner's body, as well as full involvement for both, are more important than any final outcome.

Orgasm is something more than just the simple liberation of muscular tension and subsequent relaxation: it is ecstasy. Those who practice Tantra know that reaching orgasm lets us communicate with the universe's creative power; in that moment we establish a connection with pure power, with energy.

Before we continue, let me clarify that we are not talking about just one unique orgasm because there are three different kinds of female orgasm: the clitoral, the uterine, and the mixed.

The clitoral orgasm is also known as "vaginal orgasm" and it is characterized by involuntary and rhythmic contractions of PC muscles or love muscles, and it does not require penetration to occur. Multiple orgasms and the feeling you are insatiable are common with this kind of orgasm.

The uterine orgasm is deeply emotional and it brings into play arrhythmic contractions of the PC muscles (see exercises to train them later on). Its emotional component is clearly evident because it causes an apneic response—or in other words, it temporarily stops breathing during orgasm and makes one exhale violently—while also causing other emotional reactions, such as laughter.

Regarding the uterine orgasm, it takes place following deep and fast penetrations, after reaching the cervix and the long sensitive membrane called "peritoneum," which delimits the abdomen and protects the organs, as well as the entire pelvic zone, including the uterus. This type of orgasm does not generally repeat; on the contrary, it is a single deep orgasm, and sexologists say that few women can brag about enjoying it.

Finally, the mixed orgasm combines elements from the clitoral and uterine orgasms. Normally, it is known as "vaginal orgasm" or "G-spot orgasm."

Orgasm is the definitive yield and pleasure of sex: the maximum expression that can be reached from the fusion of mind and body. It is the moment when no conflict exists, where nothing else exists: in all, the achievement and delight of the greatest pleasure.

A mixed orgasm is related to the involuntary PC muscle contractions that characterize the clitoral orgasm and is also related to deep physical and emotional satisfaction typical of the uterine orgasm. The apneic response at the orgasm's culminating moment is usually also present during the mixed orgasm. With this kind of orgasm you can enjoy multiple orgasms, although one sufficiently satisfactory orgasm is normal.

The way the PC muscles cooperate to facilitate ejaculation in the three kinds of orgasms is very interesting. In the clitoral orgasm, the vagina swells upward, while in the mixed orgasm it compresses downward making the PC muscles discharge the ejaculation to the exterior.

REMEMBER

The clitoris is sensitive because of the vulva's nerves, while the G-spot is connected to the pelvic nerves. Each causes a unique sensation of pleasure and, consequently, the respective orgasms are different. This makes it possible to experience two different types of orgasm or feel a mix of both. It always depends on the sensitivity of each of us, or of the zone we are stimulating.

THE PATH TO ORGASM...

It is a path full of pleasurable sensations that you can achieve not only with coitus, but also with many other practices, from oral sex to masturbation. But, do you know the stages your body goes through before you fully experience it? It is important that you know how to differentiate them before going into a more detailed explanation of the G-spot, ejaculation, and our *Kamasutra*.

- **Sexual arousal.** The desire that begins from the first moment, from an external stimulus. Do you remember the feeling when you passionately kiss your partner? Or how you felt that day while watching a rather suggestive movie with your partner? Or how a satisfying tingling began to run through you when, after getting home tired from work, your partner began to give you a long massage? It is the beginning of desire that runs through your whole body. In this moment your labia swell and your vulva takes on a darker color, your vagina begins to self-lubricate, and your whole body prepares for the sexual encounter.

- **The beginning of pleasure.** Although we don't realize that we enter this second stage, it takes place once foreplay has started. At this point, the first third of the vagina opens and the uterus rises slightly: it is getting ready to receive sperm. Your love muscle is flushed with blood, due to contractions that begin as a result of the waves of pleasure running through your body. It is the feeling of being "turned on." The contractions are totally involuntary and the vaginal walls become taut and taper because of them.

- **Let yourself get carried away by your senses.** We are approaching the maximum level of pleasure, the climax. Blood flows up to the breasts and you realize that they swell slightly and your nipples become hard. The clitoris is erect and hypersensitive to caresses. The vaginal labia swell. The vaginal muscles shrink and dilate in a spasmodic manner. The anus also contracts and heartbeats and breathing become progressively faster.

- **Relaxation.** You enter this stage once you have reached the orgasm, at the end of the cycle as your body recovers normal function little by little. Blood retreats from your pelvis, your chest recovers its normal rhythms, and you feel happy and relaxed. Your blood pressure decreases, your cheeks blush, and your chest shines. You have enjoyed a fully satisfactory sexual encounter!

Characteristics of the different **types of orgasm**			
	Clitoral or vaginal	**Uterine**	**Mixed or G-spot**
Feelings	Light	From light to maddening	From light to intense
Muscles	Front part of the muscles	PC and uterine muscles	Second third of PC muscles and uterine muscles
Nerves	Vulvar zone	Pelvic zone	Vulvar and pelvic zones
Techniques	Fast stimulation of clitoris	Deep penetration	G-spot stimulation
Type of ejaculation	Difficult	Possible	Easy

FIRST STEPS TO HAVING AN ORGASM

As the saying goes, "knowledge is power"; it is really important that you know what an orgasm is and what techniques and tricks you can use to reach it. Perhaps you are one of those who thinks she already knows everything about it, but if you continue reading you might discover techniques unknown to you. But you may also be one of those who doubts whether you have had one or you just feel nothing during your sexual relations... First of all, don't worry, surely it is due more to a lack of awareness of your own body than a dysfunction. Second, you can start by following this advice:

- Sexual arousal changes the ability of the genitals to feel pleasure. Foreplay and games are essential in order to enjoy fulfilling sex.

- Certain positions, such as the classic in which the man is on top of the woman (missionary position), don't produce intense sensations for a high percentage of women. The sensitive zones located in front of the vagina receive greater stimulus and satisfaction if the man positions himself behind the woman or if she is on top of him, for example. Don't forget that during coitus clitoris stimulation increases pleasure of sexual intercourse.

Finally, remember that practice is the best way to get results, and that often our own stimulation could be the most satisfying.

On the other hand, the orgasm is not just a response to a particular stimuli but also an acquired response. Thus, in order to make it a habit you just have to repeat the techniques that work best for you. Think about how you feel before and after having an orgasm, how and where do you feel it, and what are your reactions to different stimuli.

Tina Robbins, in her book *Orgasm in 5 Minutes*, summarizes this matter succinctly: "The barriers separating us from orgasm are prejudices inherited from a sexist society, in which, for centuries, female pleasure was regarded with suspicion, if not outright disapproval. Fortunately, in today's world, those prejudices are on their way out, and we women can openly reclaim the right to enjoy our bodies. All you need is some information and a bit of practice in order to enjoy an orgasm every time you make love. It doesn't matter if you are single, married, divorced, or widowed, whether you have already had sexual encounters, whether you are shy or outgoing; reaching climax will be as natural for you as eating if you are hungry or drinking when thirsty."

In both sexes, orgasm releases the sexual tension accumulated during the sexual arousal through a series of reflexive contractions, occurring mainly in the muscles surrounding the genitals.

Dare to play

After all we have covered so far, you must think that there are different stimuli to produce sexual arousal and orgasm, and you are right. These not only depend on the predisposition of the person's body, but also on external circumstances: what made you horny yesterday just by thinking about it, today might leave you cold.

I have a game for you: from the following list of types of orgasm, mark the ones you can remember having. You will see that in order to reach many of them there is no need for penetration, which increases the chances of having multiple orgasms. Do you dare to try them all? Doesn't it sound like a suggestive idea? Why don't you suggest it to your partner? Next, number the ones that you would like to have in order of preference and/or add to the list any other kinds of orgasms you might have had. The list could go on up to infinity… When you have finished reading this book and have practiced the suggested positions, ask yourself the same questions; do the answers vary?

Orgasm…
- from sexual fantasies
- while watching a pornographic movie

- with water, in the shower or bathtub
- with coitus and clitoral stimulation
- after receiving anal stimulation
- with stimulation of the whole vulva, but without penetration
- with stimulation of the labia minora and majora
- after G-spot stimulation
- with oral sex (over inner labia, outer labia, and clitoris) and without getting to penetration
- with your partner's ejaculation
- with your own ejaculation
- after receiving a massage
- only with penetration, without clitoral stimulation

Among all the previous orgasms, specialists claim that the most pleasurable one, and the one that you can repeat over and over again, is the one reached by stimulation of the G-spot, so don't skip the following pages, and exude pleasure from all the pores of your body!

A brief guide to the female sexual organs

Before we enter the fascinating world of female sexuality, and particularly the G-spot and ejaculation, it is important that you are clear about all of your sexual organs, and in order to do so you need to carefully observe your genital apparatus.

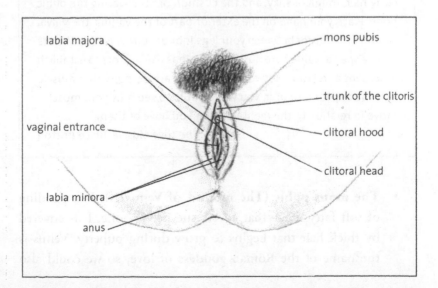

labia majora

mons pubis

trunk of the clitoris

vaginal entrance

clitoral hood

clitoral head

labia minora

anus

Unlike men's genitals, it is almost totally hidden from view, except the vulva, located in between the thighs and delimited by the mons pubis and the perineum. Pubic hair (which functions to protect the genitalia) covers, in turn, the labia majora and minora, the vaginal entrance, the clitoris, and the urethral opening. It is not uncommon that many women confess not knowing the parts of their genitalia. Nonetheless, it is important that you become familiar with them, because it is the only way to enjoy complete sexuality.

RELAX AND FIND THE MOST SECRET PARTS OF YOUR BODY

First, find a quiet place at home, where you feel comfortable. Lean back and allow yourself a moment to relax and to go over your anatomy with the help of a mirror.

"Take a mirror and lie down in your private room, naked. Do your breathing exercise and notice the tension in each part of your body. Allow your hand to rest on your legs. Notice the mons pubis, the curly hair, rough or silky, and the cushion of fat covering the pubic bone. Place your hand on the exterior part of the vagina, the vulva. Holding the mirror between your legs look at your vulva (...) Mirrors have a special value here. Just as ballerinas use mirrors to establish an essential relation between what they are doing with a muscle and the appearance of it, you will be able to see how your muscles move in relation to the mental image you have of them."

The Love Muscle, Bryce Britton

- **The mons pubis (The mound of Venus).** It is a padding of soft fatty tissue that covers the pelvic bone. It is covered by thick hair that begins to grow during puberty. Venus is the name of the Roman goddess of love, so we could also call it the "mound of love," for its fatty tissue sensitive to estrogen. It is believed that its shape is due to its function of protecting against the impact between the man and woman's pelvic bones during coitus, when penetration occurs from the front. Although at times it has been fashionable to shave pubic hair, it is not totally advisable because one of its functions is to protect the entrance of the vagina from infections and diseases.

- **Labia majora.** They are two pleats made of skin that in some cases look more like mounds and define the cleft of the vulva, covering and protecting its most delicate structures. The anterior portion of each outer lip is usually thicker than the posterior, narrowing and transitioning into the perineum. In order to explore them, lean back on the bed and carefully touch your outer lips, locating their edges. Caress them, realize how they extend from the mons pubis downward and how they form the exterior edges of the vulva. Close your eyes and let yourself get carried away with the pleasure you feel with your own caresses.

- **Labia minora.** Perhaps the most significant difference between vulvas is the size and shape of the labia minora (also called "Nymphs"). Many women have more prominent labia minora that extend beyond the labia majora. If this is not your case, don't worry at all, because it does not mean any kind of dysfunction. It is a highly erogenous zone; so much that the sexual arousal reached by caressing them is very similar to that which is achieved when caressing the clitoris.

- **Urethral opening.** It is the opening of the urethra, which allows for the passing of body fluids such as urine, female ejaculate, and the fluids of the paraurethral glands. The size and shape of the urethral opening varies considerably from one woman to another.

The urethral opening or urethral meatus can be so sensitive to sexual stimulation that it can be confused with the clitoris. Some women begin their masturbation by massaging the urethral meatus, although its stimulation through the vaginal wall is also one of the ways to ejaculate.

- **Vaginal entrance.** Shapes the mouth of the vagina (it is incorrect to refer to it as the "vaginal opening" because, unless there is something inserted in the vagina, the vaginal passage is closed). The vaginal walls are normally in contact with each other, so the vagina is a potential space, not an opening as it is normally represented. Palpate the area with one finger, introducing it into the vagina, and about a half or one inch deep you should start to feel the muscle of love, which is found suspended in between the coccyx and the pubic bone. The interior part of the vagina has a sort of canal, whose walls dilate during coitus as a response to stimulation and penetration. This canal is a humid and warm zone and the G-spot is found at its end. If you go a bit further with your finger you will feel the cervix, which is also a source of immense pleasure if it receives proper stimulation.

- **Perineum.** The flat area located between the vulvar cleft and the anus is called the perineum. It is located just below the vagina, and although many manuals state that it does not have hair, it depends on each woman. The skin of the perineum is populated with numerous nerve endings that make this zone extremely sensitive, so its stimulation produces a lot of pleasure (though it does not lead to orgasm). Due to its location, it is an area where you can receive caresses and massages during coitus.

- **The anus.** It is the opening that marks the path toward the rectum and the lower intestine, through which feces are expelled. The anal tissues are rich in blood vessels and nerve endings, so it is a highly sensitive zone, but it is also an area that requires maximum hygiene.

  Many women claim that their anus is very sensitive to stimulation and that's true. The sensitivity of this area is a protection mechanism designed to keep foreign objects out, to prevent wounds or diseases, but we can also use this response to obtain pleasure. There are many taboos about the anus; however, more and more women make it part of their sexual life every day, stimulating it with caresses or penetration. Remember that two sets of muscles surround the anus underneath the skin and that their involuntary contraction can make coitus and anal sex painful or in some cases impossible. If this happens, take your time, you should not force it. If you perform anal sex it is really important to be aware of not only the relaxation and intense sexual arousal of the participants, but also to make sure that no one feels pushed to have anal sex, because any tenseness will have painful consequences.

- **The clitoris.** It is a very complex organ and so specialized that it is the only part of the female body dedicated solely and exclusively to deliver pleasure. Until recently, it was thought that the clitoris was the only zone that could be stimulated to reach orgasm, but recent research confirms that it is not true. The clitoris consists of the same tissues as the penis and it mostly works as such; the only relevant difference between the two is that the woman's urethra does not go through the clitoral body, while in the penis it does. Men ejaculate and pass urine through the penis, while in women, although the tissues are also present, they are not connected and therefore no liquids are discharged.

Like the penis, the clitoral head is completely made of a soft erectile tissue called "corpus spongiosum." When a woman's clitoris is massaged, she experiences sexual arousal and her glans becomes more sensitive—it fills up with blood and swells. The clitoris becomes slightly bigger as if it had an erection. The size of the clitoris does not determine how sensitive it is, because the number of nerve endings does not depend on its size.

It is the most sexually sensitive part of the woman's body and it is also the easiest to stimulate. You should start slowly without rushing. Avoid touching it when dry, which is uncomfortable; first lubricate it with saliva. A word of advice: clitoral stimulation with the tip of your partner's penis is an extremely pleasurable sensation for many women. Make sure you try it.

TRY IT!

Lay down on your bed. With one hand hold the labia of the vagina wide open and with the other hand, softly caress your clitoris. The taut skin produces more intense sensations.

G-spot:
myth or reality?

A lot of literature has been dedicated to the G-spot; so much that even some specialists have questioned its existence. It is so controversial that Shere Hite refers to the "C-spot," considers the clitoris as the only organ capable of delivering pleasure and producing orgasm, and denies the importance of the G-spot. However, Aristotle had already mentioned in his writings a kind of female ejaculation, strongly linked to the existence of what we now call the G-spot. However, its existence and importance was not definitively established until the studies of Mary Jane Sherfrey, Helen Singer Kaplan, Lonnie Barbach, William H. Masters, and other physicians and sexologists of the same generation came out. These scientists carefully studied the zone that Gräfenberg described in 1950, and confirmed its existence based on surveys and the testimony of different female patients.

The G-spot used up a lot of ink in the 1970s and 1980s, both in women's magazines as well as in medical publications. But is this great sensual area of the vagina a myth or is it real? Currently, sexologists defend its existence beyond any doubt.

Years later, in 1966, Masters and Virginia Johnson also confirmed the existence of some lubricating substances secreted by the vagina that, additionally, were present in direct proportion to the woman's sexual arousal when her G-spot was stimulated. Rigorous conversations on female ejaculation began. In fact, in the majority of women the stimulation of the G-spot is connected to ejaculation, generally produced after the orgasm. Stimulation of such an area can cause intense and pleasurable sensations and not only increases the level of sexual arousal but also helps lead to orgasm.

A survey published in 1990 analyzed the relation between female ejaculation, perception of the G-spot, and the sexual arousal of 1,300 women. Its authors chose women professionally involved in health fields (physicians, nurses, psychiatrists...). Of the survey respondents, 66% noticed a special sensitivity at an indeterminate zone of the vagina that, if stimulated, produced intense pleasure different from that experienced with other zones. In those studies women stated that they believed it to be their G-spot and confessed to having ejaculations as well. Later studies on the G-spot have confirmed that its stimulation entails an increase in the perception of pleasure.

The G-spot, or Gräfenberg's spot, is a zone located at the anterior wall of the vagina, 1½ to 2 inches from the vulva. This zone, which is approximately the size of a quarter, has the capacity to bulge or swell when it is stimulated with a finger, an elongated object, or with the penis—in this last case it is reached mainly if the man is positioned behind the woman during coitus.

In 1950, Ernest Gräfenberg first described this erogenous zone. He noticed that some women have a very sensitive area on the anterior wall of their vagina, its stimulation provokes sexual arousal and pleasure, and that it reacts by swelling. At the same time, Gräfenberg discovered that the liquid evacuated through the urethra at the moment of orgasm is not urine, but a byproduct of the stimulation received. Despite all that, for a long time many women in the United States received a diagnosis of urinary incontinence due to such "leaking" of liquid during orgasm.

There is no standard size of the G-spot; it varies from one woman to another, just as we have different vulvas or arms. Thus, certain G-spots are small and when stimulated they do not enlarge as much, and vice versa. There are fat, strong ones that are easily felt in the vagina and others with little size variation that are barely perceived. However, the size does not in fact affect its response to stimulus; it depends on how sensitive to her G-spot a woman is, just as some women enjoy nipple stimulation more than others.

A DISCOVERY THAT WENT BY UNNOTICED

In the 1950s and up until the 1980s, the insensitivity of the vagina was commonly believed; only the clitoris was responsible for producing pleasure for women. The first big studies on human sexuality (the Kinsey report and the work of Masters and Johnson) had come to that conclusion, and the publication of Gräfenberg's work and conclusions were ignored until they ended up forgotten. It would have to wait until, years later, various researchers became interested in vaginal sensitivity, for his works to be taken out and dusted off once more. Perry, Whipple, and their collaborators rediscovered among many women the same phenomenon that had been described by Doctor Gräfenberg. Step-by-step, and in order to confirm this new research, new surveys were performed and different protocols were established for the G-spot to be recognized.

> The G-spot is such an important part, almost the most important, of the female sexual organ, that it is grotesque that so many women neglect it. Can you imagine if men were told they had no prostate, they do not ejaculate, and that the white liquid coming out from their penis was urine?

Before we continue our discussion, it must be said that prior to being scientifically recognized, this spot seems to have gained a mythical place in the sexual imaginations of both men and women: "The zone whose stimulation produces pleasures never even dreamed of!" "Find your G-spot or your partner's and you will discover sensations never felt before!" "Orgasm almost immediately by stimulating the G-spot!" And in fact, the authors of these statements were not wrong...

Locate and stimulate your G-spot

Now that the preliminaries are taken care of, we can dive into the main topic: the G-spot. I will begin by telling you that finding the G-spot is not an easy task if you don't know exactly where it is, which explains why some women end up believing that they don't have one. Those who have in fact found it claim to enjoy the sexual act in positions in which the man is on top, doggy style, or the savage furor, because these allow better contact between the penis and the front wall of the vagina, where the spot is located (see a description and explanation of these positions later). Firm pressure, a fast pace, and a lot of friction will achieve the goal of the G-spot orgasm. It is curious how many women have a sensation similar to the need to urinate when stimulation first begins, so we recommend you use the bathroom before beginning to make love. Although you may ejaculate—discharge a small amount of a white or transparent liquid when you reach climax—it has nothing to do with urine.

Perhaps, your partner and you will struggle a bit to find the magic G-spot, but it is worth trying. It is worthwhile because with its stimulation you both can reach intense new sensations.

As we have seen, the G-spot's location is about the same in all women, with slight variations; for some it is located in the anterior wall of the vagina, while for others their posterior wall is the most sensitive to stimuli. However, we are often unable to describe with accuracy and precision the exact place where all kinds of intense "emotions" are produced.

Silvia de Béjar, in *Tu sexo es tuyo* (*Your Sex Is Yours*), explains a very useful trick in order to locate it: "Imagine that you have a clock in the interior of your vagina where noon is pointing in the direction of your belly button. You should search for your G-spot between eleven and one o'clock. The pressure on this zone is what stimulates the urethral sponge, which has numerous nerve endings and blood vessels that, when stimulated, produce pleasure."

If you want to discover your G-spot on your own, you'd better find a comfortable place at home and commit to exploring your body carefully; it is the only way you will end up finding it, and can begin to enjoy caressing it. Once you have located it, you can turn to a vibrator for help in stimulating it if you want. There are ones that are made specifically for the G-spot.

Now I will explain in more detail the steps that you can follow in order to find your G-spot, but keep in mind that it is not an easy task—though certainly not impossible—and don't forget that you will find it easier if you are aroused, because it swells and stands out more with sexual arousal. Don't worry or get obsessed if you can't find it in the first few attempts—that won't stop you from having a healthy sex life or enjoying it. While locating and stimulating it, if you feel like urinating, even though you emptied your bladder beforehand, don't be alarmed. This is normal; you are very likely ejaculating already (see the chapter "Another look at female pleasure: ejaculation"). Now, let's find our G-spot!

How to find your G-spot

As you can see in the illustration of the female sexual organs, the tissue surrounding the urethra covers the G-spot. It is not always easy to locate and stimulate it with your hand, so it might be more pleasurable to do it with a special vibrator (we will talk more about this later). But now, without further preamble, carefully read the following steps:

1. Sit quietly, relax, and get ready to locate the three central zones of your vagina. Don't forget that if you lie down face up it is more complicated, because gravity tends to push the internal organs down and, consequently, farther from the vaginal entrance. The best position is seated or crouching down, so sit on the ground over a towel and bring a mirror. Locate your clitoris and determine its distance from the entrance of your vagina. Next, locate the urinary meatus

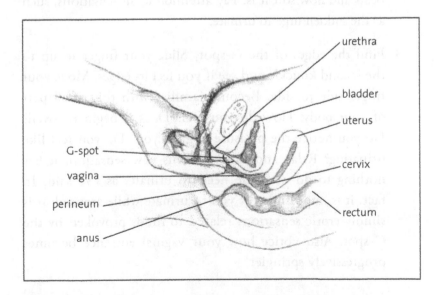

and notice its distance from the clitoris and the vaginal entrance. This will help you to correctly visualize your sexual organs, as well as the clitoral stimulation that you can receive during penetration.

2. Look at the movements of your urethral opening. If you want, use a vibrator (always lubricating it beforehand). Insert it in your vagina and notice the movements of your urinary meatus. Does it get closer to or farther from the vibrator? Change the vibrator's angle and see if your meatus changes position. If it is a finger width apart, it will be more difficult to ejaculate with something inserted in the vagina, because of the pressure exerted on the urethra. Take out the vibrator. With a finger, touch your urinary meatus and the spongy area surrounding it. Slowly introduce the finger into your vagina about up to the first knuckle, pressing it upward lightly. Notice how the urethra is connected with the vagina, how it beats and how soft it is. Pay attention to all sensations, such as the sudden urge to urinate.

3. Find the edges of the G-spot. Slide your finger in up to the second knuckle and see if you feel its edges. Move your finger side to side. Become familiar with this small part of your body. How do you feel? Does it begin to swell? Do you notice the pleasure it gives you? Do you feel like urinating? Relax and focus on this new sensation; it has nothing to do with the need to urinate, as I've said. In fact, it is impossible for you to urinate while aroused; it is simply erotic sensations related to fluids provoked by the G-spot. Also notice how your vaginal entrance becomes progressively springier.

4. Insert one or two fingers into the vagina and imagine there is a kind of egg that is partially leaning against the bottom wall of the vagina. Slowly move your finger around this imaginary egg, feel the edges with detail, and caress it. The part that has swollen and beats strongly is, undoubtedly, your G-spot.

5. Feel your G-spot with all its strength. Move your finger around the area in which your G-spot is located. Go over the whole area soothingly and meticulously, entertain yourself with it, reaching as far as the cervix (don't worry if you have to stick your finger all the way in to do so). Bend your finger upward and slightly left; this finger position is very important because it facilitates G-spot location and stimulation. Notice how your G-spot swells, how it beats, how it begins to give you pleasure.

6. Now, all that's left is to get an approximate idea of its size; take advantage of this to enjoy your own caresses.

STEPS TO LOCATE YOUR G-SPOT

1. Locate the different parts of your sexual organs.
2. Look at the movements of the urinary meatus.
3. Feel your urethral zone.
4. Find your G-spot's margins.
5. Notice its size and how it swells.
6. Locate its ending point.
7. Explore how the tissue feels.
8. Note how your PC muscles contract and make you throb with pleasure.

ENJOY LOCATING THE G-SPOT WITH YOUR PARTNER

The second time I made love with Alejandro, he made sure to look for my G-spot (I had tried finding it before without any luck); in order to do so he inserted his fingers inside me and softly palpated my interior until I felt a great arousal and he, in turn, had the sensation of being in contact with something different. I had a different kind of orgasm, intense and deep. Later, while he was stimulating the G-spot, he did the same with my clitoris... Don't hesitate to experiment until you find it: it is like touching the sky.

Cecilia, 41 years old

If you have a partner with whom you feel comfortable, you will want to share the discovery of your G-spot with him or her. In order to do so, the best technique is to lie facedown on the bed with your legs spread apart and hips slightly lifted. Tell your partner to introduce two fingers, with their palm facing down, and to explore the anterior wall of your vagina with some pressure. It will be closer to the bed. Move your pelvis to help your partner make contact with the G-spot and be sure to give feedback on the sensations of pleasure you are experiencing as he introduces his fingers and moves them slowly but without stopping.

Let's locate it in a different position. This time position yourself facing up and have your partner introduce two fingers very gently into your vagina, but now with their palm facing up. You will feel the G-spot by pressing against the superior wall of the vagina, located halfway between the back of the pubic bone and where the vagina joins the cervix. Tell your partner to rest the other hand on your abdomen, about where your pubic hair begins, and apply light pressure downward; this contributes to a greater stimulation of the G-spot and your pleasure will increase considerably.

REACHING THE SUPREME PLEASURE

Now you know where your G-spot is. Don't forget that it is a very sensitive zone that you must treat carefully and gently. The first steps will help you to locate it and to feel its extreme sensitivity. Don't forget that, no matter the method you use to stimulate it, you need to be sexually aroused, because that will allow for vaginal lubrication and the insertion of an object.

If oral sex is not part of your foreplay, now is a good time to change that habit and get to know some different sensations. You can also stimulate yourself by caressing the clitoris with your fingers before your partner enters your vagina.

There are three highly recommended techniques that you can try with a partner in order to stimulate the G-spot:

- **Stimulation with hand.** In order to stimulate the G-spot manually, have your partner place his or her finger softly and rhythmically on the spot. This type of caress requires a lot of tact and rapport between the two of you, because your partner can speed up or slow down the rhythm according to your needs and increase or reduce pressure depending on your indications, in order to change the degree of your arousal.

  I advise before performing these kind of caresses that your hands are totally clean and nails well trimmed; it would not hurt if you both start with some cream or lubricant to make it easier the first time you try it. The sensations you have could be less intense than those of the clitoral orgasm but you will be able to reach orgasm faster and repeatedly. This is favorable because you can also combine it with clitoral stimulation or stimulation of other erogenous zones.

- **Stimulation with penis.** This could be difficult if there hasn't been enough arousing foreplay to make your vagina well lubricated. Due to its position and the natural shape of the penis, the best positions to stimulate this zone are those in which the woman places herself on top of the man or she is penetrated from behind (see the positions of our *Kamasutra*).

- **Stimulation with sexual objects.** Many women experience a lot of pleasure by inserting objects in their vagina or anus. The object should be soft, not excessively rigid, and it must be very clean before using it. If possible, the object can be covered with a condom and adequately lubricated. You can use a variety of objects: from sex toys such as dildos or vibrators, to phallic fruits and vegetables in the shape of a penis, small plastic bottles, rolled up clothes, etc. Imagination is the best tool in these cases. Here are a few ideas:
  - You can set up your own homemade vibrator by placing a damp towel over an electric toothbrush or using the side of your electric shaving machine.
  - Place your turned-on vibrator on the bed. Spread your legs and lay facing down over it.
  - Kneel on the bed and bring your head to the pillow. Insert a vibrator in your vagina or anus.
  - Place a towel between your legs. Press your legs together or cross one over the other. Slide the towel against the clitoris rhythmically.
  - Place the edge of a towel between your legs and lie face-down on the bed. Without using your hands and just with forceful movement of your hips and legs, rub the towel over your vulva, especially over the clitoris.

The vibrator is the modern version of the dildo, and has become the most popular sex toy. In fact, many people regard it as the best sex toy. There is a wide range of vibrators on the market: models with special accessories for clitoral stimulation; anal vibrators with a protector to prevent them from staying inside; and even small egg-shaped vibrators that are meant to be inserted in the vagina. And, of course, vibrators that, because of their curved shape, are designed to better access the G-spot.

The most modern vibrators spin and move with the help of a mechanism, and come with different heads to modify sensations and rhythms. These powerful, trusty vibrators are also sold as body massagers. However, don't fool yourself— they're no match for the strong and consistent stimulation applied by your or your partner's own hand.

Next, you will see the most commonly used ones; you can select which of them you think can best fulfill your needs. Although the use of vibrators and dildos has not always been well accepted, my advice is that you don't let yourself be influenced by those old-fashioned beliefs and take advantage of everything you can to get the greatest pleasure possible. The only thing you have to watch out for is hygiene; the rest is up to you—and your partner, if you use them as a couple.

- **Dildos.** The dildo is simply an artificial penis that can help you reach orgasm with good sexual stimulation. They are good for both anal and vaginal insertion. They don't vibrate, and if you don't move them, they do nothing. These devices may be made of different materials, such as silicone, wood, stainless steel, etc. The most modern version of these dildos are the vibrators.

- **Vibrators with a wand and accessories.** A vibrator with a wand produces a diffused and penetrating sensation. Its flexible head is joined to a handle, which allows a lot of maneuverability during penetration. It adapts well to the couple in many different positions.

- **Vibrators with cables and accessories.** Wired vibrators have a lot of followers. They are smaller and the vibrations are focused and extremely fast. Also they are not noisy. They include a set of accessories that could be used for external stimulation.

Now you can act: "A little bit deeper, baby." As you will see, it's not difficult to manually stimulate the G-spot. The best way is, once you both are aroused with a bit of slow and gentle foreplay, for the man to slide his finger into the vagina once it's wet enough. He should do it with care along the upper wall of the vagina, until he notices the rounded shape of the G-spot, which will be a little bit more swollen. Once it's located he should press it softly and go over it with his fingers slowly, giving a soft massage to increase your pleasure.

You can repeat this technique as many times as you both want, thinking only about pleasure. If you don't feel anything, take your time and ask your partner to keep on massaging; you probably need a longer period of stimulation for you to get the arousing effect and desired sensations.

THE BEST SEXUAL POSITIONS

There are many positions for sex that enable the penis to reach the G-spot. Would you like to know about them and enjoy the most intimate secrets with your partner?

WOMAN ON TOP

"I have always liked to be on top in all my sexual practices. This position feels a little kinkier and establishes a domination dynamic between us that satisfies us more than others. Besides, in this position Fernando always reaches my G-spot with his penis and I have multiple orgasms."

Marina, 28 years old

In this position the woman places herself on top of the man facing away from him, seated, or lying down. This position allows for caresses in all erogenous zones of the woman's body while penetration takes place. Also, the man has easy access to his partner's anus and buttocks, and she can slow down her movements to enjoy anal stimulation or caresses over her breasts.

The slant of this posture creates an angle that allows the man's penis to directly hit the G-spot. Whether you are a woman who can reach orgasm easily with this stimulation, or one who has not located the G-spot, this kind of penetration is always the most satisfying.

Furthermore, since the man is comfortably lying down, it seems like he is just waiting to receive pleasure as his partner wishes, which you may find sexy. You both can take advantage of this game of masculine submission as another stimulant: the encounter can start by giving him kisses and caresses, as he remains in the same position, and then finish with a deep penetration. The woman controls the movement with her arms and can increase the eroticism by looking at her partner over her shoulder and pretending to be unreachable.

If the woman leans her whole body backward, and rests her arms on her partner's, she can also extend her legs forward to increase the angle. This way the man can easily reach her breasts during moments of ecstasy and the woman will be able to rest her buttocks on her partner's belly and make circular movements to guide the penis toward the G-spot, enjoying the moment of great eroticism and sensuality.

MAN ON TOP

"It is a different experience from any other that I have ever had with a man. Alberto and I can lie down facing each other and his penis reaches that part of my vagina that causes a really amazing orgasm. I think it is due to the position of the penis

when erect, pushed against his belly. I had never experienced
such pleasurable sensations!

Ana, 37 years old

This position could work better or worse depending on the G-spot's location and the size and shape of the penis. A man with a spur-shaped penis will surely reach his partner's G-spot without any trouble. When you do it the man should apply a slow and rhythmic pressure, never rough or sudden. You can also place a pillow under the woman's hips, so the vagina is at the proper angle.

REMEMBER

"G-spot stimulation is related not only to the position selected for the sexual act, but also to the physical configuration and the cooperation of the couple's members. Gräfenberg told us something more about the man's role: the angle between the member and the body is of great importance and must be kept in mind. It is possible that the legend of the ideal lover is based on these physiological characteristics."

Ladas and Whipple in their book *El punto G y otros descubrimientos recientes sobre sexualidad* (*The G-spot and Other Recent Findings on Sexuality*)

ON THE SIDE

"It was hard at first to position myself not facing my partner to make love; there were many taboos in my mind about anal sex. However, one day I decided to try it. From then on my best orgasms come when I am penetrated from behind. That is when I can guide my partner for real towards the proper spot and help him reach with his penis the exact spot to bring me to orgasm."

Luisa, 42 years old

In the lateral position, the woman is normally penetrated from behind, for which she must place her upper leg on top of her partner. There is also a little variant in which she stretches a leg backward and wraps it around his waist. The woman lies on her side and the man positions himself behind her back to penetrate her. That allows the man to have more room for penetration to reach the front wall of the vagina consistently and firmly so the G-spot is being stimulated. Since this position doesn't allow for much movement, it is easy for the man to maintain penetration for longer and the woman can adjust the pressure on her vaginal wall by flexing her hips back or raising her leg. It is ideal for gifted men and flexible women and fulfills several common fantasies: first of all, the fact that her back is facing him could simulate anal coitus and, at the same time, the man can reach her face and neck. This position also allows comfortable access to the clitoris and breasts. The opening of her legs to receive the penis and the hug of that same leg around her partner is perhaps the most pleasurable part of this position, which will make you reach unforgettable orgasms. Be sure to try it out!

FROM BEHIND

"The first time my husband asked me to let my body fall forward, offering him my butt and relaxing myself, I wasn't sure that I would enjoy it. Now, I admit that it is the best position for me to orgasm. I think it's because his penis can better stimulate my G-spot."

Margarita, 32 years old

This sex position is ideal for lovers who want the most impudent and wildest sex. Penetration from behind is particularly suggested for women who have given birth, because their nervous zones are much more "alert" and are much more sensitive to stimulation. Since the vaginal canal is more flexible, the penis can easily reach the desired zone, the G-spot. Keep in mind that a woman on all fours can lower her shoulders to increase the angle of pressure and increase the pleasure for both herself and her partner during penetration. Since the man is standing, he takes the woman from behind and penetrates her by holding her by the waist. Meanwhile, the woman has relaxed her body and lets it fall until her hands are resting on the floor. Then the man "surprises" her from behind and sets the rhythm of the coitus—first slowly, then finishing stronger and reaching orgasm after stimulating her G-spot. For her, the pleasure is concentrated in the angle of her vaginal entrance that, since it is constricted by this position, causes a sensation of tightness and is very pleasurable for many women and usually leads to orgasm. For him, the strongest sensation comes from the glans, which enters and exits the vagina as he pleases, even caressing the clitoris at times, provoking an even greater arousal. In his field of vision is her anus, buttocks, and back, highly erogenous zones for many, which he can caress while penetrating her. His domination and her total relaxation can favor anal play: introducing a finger during coitus can be enormously arousing and pleasurable, and may lead you to the most satisfying orgasms.

STANDING, SEATED, OR KNEELING DOWN

"The truth is that it came to us almost by chance when Victor grabbed me by the back of the knees. It was one of those days that we decided to try out new positions in bed, just for the fun of trying. Now I know that this is the position to repeat because it guarantees me an orgasm."

Alicia, 48 years old

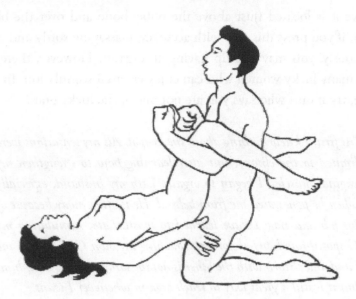

In this posture the man must remain kneeling or standing while he penetrates his partner at a 90° angle, which ensures that he will reach her G-spot. She lies face up on the bed and places her heels on her partner's shoulders or her legs over his elbows. Either position allows both partners to guide the penis to their preferred angle. In this position he can show off his work at the gym by bending his arms and holding her with his strength. The more he pulls up the woman's hips, the greater the pressure on the G-spot and the better orgasms his partner will enjoy.

ORGASM THROUGH G-SPOT STIMULATION

We already know that the G-spot is an area of maximum sensitivity where stimulation can produce one or many orgasms, but the most surprising thing is that, according to some sexologists, it is also possible to reach orgasm by pressing the G-spot from the exterior.

Once it is located (just above the pubic bone and over the bladder), if you press this area with accuracy, massaging softly and continuously, you may end up having an orgasm. However, there are not many lucky women who can enjoy external stimulation. In any case, try it out; who says you are not one of the lucky ones?

> *"At first, I knew nothing about the G-spot. All my sensations were limited to the clitoris, but after learning how to strengthen my vaginal muscles, I began to orgasm with my husband, especially when he penetrated me from behind. He is often away because of his job and now I have learned to masturbate, stimulating my G-spot through my abdomen. Touching my own G-spot with one hand and clitoris with the other is not the same as being with him, but it is still a great way to reach orgasm whenever I want."*

Testimony gathered from Ladas and Whipple in their book *El punto G y otros descubrimientos sobre sexualidad* (*The G-spot and Other Findings on Sexuality*).

Are you one of those women who feel nothing? If you are one of those women who say you don't feel anything from G-spot stimulation, or you simply believe you don't have one, let your partner know. It could be a good idea to have him help you find it and estimate its size during foreplay. Ask him to move his fingers from the mouth of the vagina to where it meets the G-spot. You can try it before you are aroused and then repeat it later; that way you both will realize how the size of the G-spot has changed. It is really useful to talk about what is going on and what you are feeling as he caresses you. If the woman feels that the pleasurable sensations increase with the massage it means that everything is on the right track. From then on it's about the sensations progressively leading toward orgasm. However, if you don't feel any increase of size, or don't feel anything special, you will not reach orgasm or ejaculate, which can be due to various reasons:

1. G-spot stimulation has not been accurate or has been too brief.
2. You are not aroused enough to make your G-spot swell and reach orgasm.
3. You may be part of the 10% of women who have a too-small G-spot or one located deeper in the vagina, which makes it harder to access.

In any case, the only thing you shouldn't do is worry. Worrying makes sexual relations more difficult because it tenses the muscles. Perhaps it is more about being relaxed and letting yourself get carried away, without feeling self-conscious. And remember: practice helps to improve sexuality.

Strengthen your PC muscles

In 1947, gynecologist Arnold Kegel, concerned about the number of women suffering from urinary incontinence, began research that led him to invent a device—Kegel's perineometer—for the strengthening of pelvic muscles and thus avoiding leaking of urine. The woman would introduce the device into her vagina and it would contract her pelvic muscles. It concerned the area that was located at the end of the PC muscles, the muscles of love, greatly responsible for orgasms because they facilitate stimulation of the G- and K-spots (see explanation of the K-spot later).

Kegel also designed a set of exercises that were meant for women suffering from urinary incontinence; it was later observed that if these women practiced them, they had much more pleasurable relations and more intense orgasms.

LOCATE THE LOVE MUSCLE

The first step to perform Kegel's exercises is to locate the love muscle, the pubococcygeus, or PC muscle. While you are urinating, try to stop the stream and let it go again, contracting and dilating the muscle. It is important to spread your legs so the buttocks don't interfere in the exercise. Don't use this technique as a daily practice while you urinate, because you could end up getting an infection; just use it to locate the muscle. Don't worry if you can't get it on the first attempt; relax and start over again. Contract and relax, focusing on the sensation and visualizing the muscle in your interior.

Insert a finger inside your vagina and press it without contracting the muscles in your legs. The important thing is that you notice how the love muscle contracts. As you can see in the illustration, the muscle is surrounded by others, but it is the most important one in the pelvis and you will be able to identify it among them. And what is even more important, you will soon discover its benefits.

According to Kegel, a PC muscle that is in good shape can be as wide as three fingers, while a weak one could be as thin as a pencil. If you palpate your vaginal wall, every half inch you get deeper on it, you should be able to notice the muscle. You should even realize when it compresses. After performing the test with only one finger, try doing it with two. Insert two fingers, one next to the other, as deep as you can. Then, separate those fingers as if they were a pair of scissors and try to force your fingers back together by strongly contracting the PC muscles. If you can do it, congratulations! If not, don't worry, you will get it later; you just have to keep reading this book.

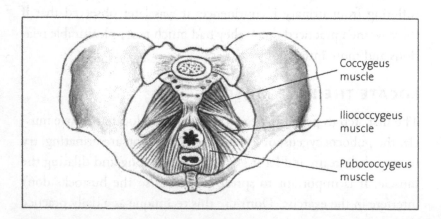

Coccygeus muscle

Iliococcygeus muscle

Pubococcygeus muscle

When a woman is able to control the love muscle she will undoubt-edly reach orgasms never experienced before. If a man exercises this muscle and prepares, he will have better control of his ejaculation.

DO YOU KNOW HOW TO CALCULATE THE STRENGTH OF YOUR PC MUSCLES?

Before resuming, and if you have not been able to successfully complete the previous exercise, it's best to calculate the flexibility and resistance of your PC muscle. Again, insert one or more fingers in your vagina, wetting them with saliva or lubricant before you start. I suggest you perform this test many times, before and after reading the exercises to strengthen them, explained later, and you will notice the improvement. Now, answer the following questions to assess the condition of your PC muscles:

- The mouth of my vagina is very elastic and it stretches and contracts as soon as I introduce my finger, but I cannot contract my muscles.

- The mouth of my vagina is very elastic and it stretches and contracts as soon as I introduce my finger, and I notice some pressure from the muscles.

- The entrance of my vagina is very elastic and stretches and contracts; also, my vaginal muscles hold my finger firmly.

- The mouth of my vagina is really tight, but I can introduce one finger. Then I rest it on the vaginal walls, toward the anus, and I feel how it relaxes.

- The entrance of my vagina is too tight for me to introduce a finger.

CAUSES OF PC MUSCLES WEAKENING

- **Pregnancy:** because of the weight of the uterus.
- **Labor:** after the baby passes through the vagina.
- **Post-labor:** premature exercising of abdominal muscles or jumping, practicing a sport, or carrying too much weight.
- **Sports:** especially the ones involving "jumping," or "impact" sports.
- **Menopause:** because of the hormonal changes; they cause a loss of elasticity, atrophy, and hypotony.
- **Heredity:** two in every ten women have innate weakness in the pelvic floor muscles.
- **Daily habits:** retaining urine, wearing very tight clothes, practicing singing, and playing wind instruments.
- **Other causes:** obesity, constipation, chronic cough, stress, and others.

Exercises to strengthen the PC muscle. There are different exercises that will help us strengthen and control these muscles. As a general rule, the better shape they are in, the greater the pleasure will be during sexual relations. Luckily, just like all muscles of the body, the PC can be trained with proper exercises.

A loose and untrained muscle has little sensitivity, while a healthy muscle is more sensitive to physical stimulation and, therefore, provides pleasure. Thus, correct practice of Kegel's exercises, based on continued and brief contractions of the pubococcygeus muscle, alternated with relaxation periods, will give you the muscular resistance and sensitivity needed to improve your sexual practices.

- **Slow exercise.** Tighten the muscles just like you did when you tried to stop the urine stream, as if you were pulling them upward. Contract and keep them like that while you count to five, breathing softly, relaxed. Then, relax them for five more seconds, and repeat the series ten times. Try to progressively increase the intervals of contraction and relaxation. Begin with five seconds each up to twenty. The longer you can hold the muscles, the stronger they will become.

- **Fast exercise.** Tighten and relax the muscles as fast as you can until you get tired or for about two to three minutes (whichever happens first). Start with a series of ten repetitions four times per day until you get to fifty daily repetitions.

- **Combined exercise.** Contract the PC muscle combining short and long intervals, ten times in total. Repeat a maximum of three times per session.

- **Squeezing exercise.** Contract the PC muscle as long as possible before relaxing it. Try to get two minutes.

- **The elevator.** This exercise requires some focus, but its results are very good. Your vagina is a muscular tube with ring-shaped sections set one over another. Imagine that each of the sections is a different floor of a building, to which you go up and down in an elevator, and you apply tension in each section. Begin by lifting the elevator up to the first floor, hold it for one second, and go to the next floor. Keep on going up as many floors as you can (normally not more than five). To go down, also hold for a second at each "floor." When you get to the lower part, try to go to the basement, pushing the pelvic muscles downward for a few seconds (just like if you were in labor). Last, try a total relaxation of the muscles for a few seconds. It is important that you don't forget to breathe slowly and that you avoid aiding yourself with the abdominal muscles to perform the exercises.

• **If you are a woman.** Insert a finger in your vagina and contract your PC muscle.

• **The wave.** Some of the muscles from the pelvic floor are set up following a figure-eight pattern, but with three rings. One ring is located around the urethra, a second is around the vagina, and the last one is around the anus. Contract these muscles from front to back and relax them from back to front. Perform these exercises as many times as you can per day. The goal is to perform them without others realizing. When you begin to practice, they can seem weird, but soon you will see how you can carry them out while people around don't even notice. At first, when practicing the slow exercise, you may notice that the muscles resist remaining contracted; it's also possible that you get tired after the fast exercise. However, if you persist, you will see that in a few days they will not take any effort at all.

"Having powerful muscles and exercising them during sex helps achieve orgasm for those women that don't have them, improve orgasms for those that do have them, and help women have more. It also benefits the penis stimulation."

Lorena Berdú, *Nuestro Sexo (Our Sex)*

• **Squeezing slowly and continuously.** This exercise is perhaps the most commonly practiced by women because it compresses and holds the muscle in a prolonged contraction. You have to start with three seconds of contraction and gradually increase the time until you get a contraction of ten seconds. When you finish the contraction, relax the muscle entirely and start over again. Contract and gradually tighten until you increase resistance. You will notice how the vaginal walls get closer and farther, which is what increases your and your partner's pleasure at the moment of penetration.

- **Stretch and loosen.** This is the ideal exercise to tone the whole pelvic area; it also stimulates vaginal lubrication and strengthens the vaginal and uterine muscles, which in turn will have an effect on your enjoyment during coitus. To do it, lift the upper part of your pelvis, with help from your abdominal muscles, as well as the love muscle. My advice is that you practice it in the morning while in bed. The exercise consists of three parts that might last from five to ten seconds. Start by breathing deeply while you contract the love muscle and then, for about three seconds, pull upward from the lower part of the pelvis, as if you had a tampon inside the vaginal canal and you were preventing it from falling out. If you focus you will feel the vaginal walls surrounding it. Now contract the muscle and perform a movement like if you wanted to aspirate the tampon upward. (It is not advisable to introduce anything in your vagina during this exercise because it can be dangerous). Then hold that position for a few seconds and pull inward between two and five seconds (it will depend on your skill level) and keep the imaginary tampon inside the vagina. Last, push it out as if you wanted the tampon to get out on its own.

- **Beats.** Do you feel your heart beating? Well, in this exercise your beat is what is going to tell you when to loosen and relax your love muscle following its rhythm. If at first it's hard for you to follow your heart rate, take a break and do it with every other beat, or every three or four beats. With some patience you will learn to follow your heart rate. With this exercise you will increase the resistance of your love muscles, and this seems to be the key step for reaching orgasm.

Do not repeat the exercises more often than instructed, because, like all muscular exercises, they can make the muscles sore, or you can end up with cramps. After a few days of practice you can go ahead and perform more than one session per day, but not before.

If, after performing these exercises, you notice a backache or pain in the abdominal muscles, it's because you are doing them incorrectly. Try to properly locate the PC muscle and work only with this muscle.

TRAINING YOUR LOVE MUSCLE

The ideal would be that right now, while you are reading, you tightened your love muscle and felt the satisfaction of creating and controlling your own orgasm. Here are guidelines for training and strengthening the love muscle:
1. Squeezing slowly and continuously
2. Stretch and loosen
3. Beats

After practicing exercises on a regular basis for a few weeks, you can repeat the "scissors" test or check on how you are controlling the urine stream. Do you notice any difference from your first attempts? Don't worry if the changes are small; in a few days you will notice some more little improvements.

And remember, as Tina Robbins affirms in her book *Orgasm in 5 Minutes*: "It will require a little extra concentration only at the beginning. Then everything will be a breeze and you can practice anywhere because nobody will notice. You can do it while lying, standing, sitting, or reclined. On the bus, at work, leaning at a bar: only you will be aware that you are contracting and relaxing the muscles of your vagina and preparing to fully enjoy sex... when the time comes."

Men's PC muscle

Just like women, men have a PC muscle that, if they know how to control it, is a good ally to control erection and ejaculation. This muscle is located above the perineum and if the man can relax and contract it at will, it not only helps him control ejaculation and erection but also improves blood flow and muscle tone of the genitalia. Sexologists suggest exercising the contraction and relaxation of the muscle throughout the day as a way to overcome problems derived from male sexuality. Furthermore, recent research studies confirm that men are as capable as women of experiencing multiple orgasms and that, most likely, controlling and training the pubococcygeus muscles is the most important factor in doing so.

The PC muscle can be located easily. When the man is urinating he can find it by contracting and relaxing the muscle that stops the stream of urine. If he wants to visually locate it, its contraction can be observed in front of the mirror; even when the penis is not erect, if he has sufficient strength in the PC muscles he can easily lift it up.

With diligent practice of these exercises, it's possible to not just improve the erection but also make it last longer. In the case of ejaculation, when the muscle is contracted the flow of blood to the spongy tissue of the penis is cut off and he can control it as long as he wishes. This technique can be very pleasurable during coitus, because the man can extend his pleasure while being inside of his partner's vagina and until she reaches orgasm.

One of the most successful exercises in terms of its outcome is the towel test. A man with strong pubococcygeus muscles is able to hang a small towel on his erected member. If the muscles are weak he can start by trying it with a handkerchief.

Another look at female pleasure: ejaculation

"For some time now, I know that women ejaculate because of my own personal experience. I used to feel disturbed by it, but I always knew it was something natural and that the liquid I was discharging was not urine. Compared to other kinds of orgasm, the one that produces ejaculation causes a sensation of more complete withdrawal. And, although the experience is deeper than that of the usual orgasm, it turns out to be easier to become aroused again." This is one of the many examples that Ladas and Whipple offer us in their book *El punto G y otros descubrimientos recientes sobre sexualidad* (*The G-spot and Other Findings on Sexuality*), and it confirms the existence of female ejaculation.

The sexologists' studies were right, although they were not the first ones to discuss this topic. It is possible to find references to the liquids that women discharge during sexual relations in the *Kamasutra*, the Chinese sexual manuals of the Yellow Emperor, the writings of Hippocrates, and even in Aristotle's texts. And it was precisely this "liquid," usually mistaken for urine because it is so copious that it can end up soaking the bed, that led the majority of sexologists to confirm the existence of the G-spot.

> When the muscular contractions in the vagina's surroundings are vigorous enough to make an orgasm happen, some viscous substances are expelled from the vagina, and this is what is known as "female ejaculation."

Female ejaculation is a sensual and fun phenomenon that takes place when the woman is aroused. The sensation it produces is infinitely liberating and erotic. However, not every woman ejaculates spontaneously; sometimes it takes some training that requires no more than a clear knowledge of the female anatomy, because ejaculation is an innate phenomenon.

Forget the clichés that claim that the majority of women do not ejaculate; they usually go along with the denial of the G-spot as well. The truth is that all of us, all women, are born with the anatomic ability to ejaculate, just like we are born with arms, feet, a nose, or ears; we just need to know the tricks in order to learn how to do it. As Ladas and Whipple put it in their book *El punto G y otros descubrimientos recientes sobre sexualidad* (*The G-spot and Other Findings on Sexuality*): "We take for granted that all women have a G-spot and all men have a prostate gland. Their function to some extent depends on the condition of the surrounding muscles. Almost all men ejaculate, as well as many women, and we emphasize one more time that the process of ejaculation is directly affected by the condition of the muscles involved in the process."

The fact that some women ejaculate at the moment of orgasm has been, like many other aspects of female sexuality, condemned to silence by the dominant morals. However, female ejaculation, far from being something esoteric or secondary, is a very important part of women's sexuality. Although not every woman ejaculates, it doesn't prevent them from having a healthy sex life. Other women ejaculate spontaneously after reaching orgasm and some have learned how to do it.

> In 1950, Gräfenberg observed that some women discharged great amounts of a clear liquid from the urethra during orgasm. And he thought that the liquid was secreted by the intraurethral glands. In 1978, J. Lowndes and Dr. Bennet came to the conclusion that some women ejaculate and the source of such ejaculation is the "female prostate," a system of glands and pipes that enclose the female urethra and develops from the same embryological tissue as the male prostate.

"Over the years I have experienced ejaculation very often. It has been a stream of liquid abundant enough to soak the bed and different from lubrication, with a characteristic smell. It normally happens when my husband penetrates me from behind, but it also happens in other positions. Far from being uncomfortable, my husband and I have always linked this phenomenon with a much more intense pleasure. And the truth is that it has usually come with multiple orgasms for both parties."

Maria, 38 years old

In some cases, the so-called "female ejaculation" is produced by a spontaneous reflex of the vaginal production area. To achieve this, all you need is stimulation of the proper place. This place is located in the anterior face of the vagina, halfway between the pubic bone and the cervix, about one inch from the vagina's exterior: the G-spot. Indeed, this zone—capable of producing an erection in its tissues similar to the male glans—is also capable of secreting a whitish and odorless substance similar to the one produced in the male prostate, on top of being a source of great sexual satisfaction. This transparent liquid has a consistency similar to the one of a light lubricant, more aqueous than viscous, with an odor and flavor that varies depending on where you are in your menstrual cycle. Although it has not been proven, it seems that this substance is expelled by pressure through the urethra after it has built up in the so called "periurethral glands," embryologically related to the male prostate, which are located in Gräfenberg's zone. Therefore, it has nothing to do with urination but a lot to do with the G-spot. Gräfenberg additionally linked production of this liquid directly to the orgasm (although you can also produce it without reaching orgasm, as I'll explain to you later): "This spasmodic expulsion of liquid always occurs in the crucial moment of the orgasm and coincides with it. If there is a chance to observe these women's orgasm, it is possible to see that great amounts of a clear and transparent liquid is expelled in streams not through the vulva but the urethra. The profuse secretions that come with the orgasm do not have any lubricating purpose, otherwise they would take place at the beginning of the sexual act and not during the final moments of the orgasm."

Nevertheless, and although female ejaculation and its mysteries require confidence and commitment to working out your body's response, the outcome will confirm that all your work has been worthwhile.

Never forget this crucial point: practice safe sex. There are no studies related to the transmission of diseases from the ejaculation, so you have to be extremely careful. Since female ejaculate exits the same pipe that men's sperm does and since, unlike men, you have no way of containing it with a condom, I advise you refrain if you or your partner have any sexually transmitted diseases.

EJACULATE MANUALLY

Once you have located your G-spot, you will have discovered how sexual relations can become much more pleasurable than you previously imagined. The next step is an advanced technique to ejaculate manually. Once you have enough knowledge about stimulation of your G-spot and awareness of its swelling, you can make it ejaculate. Your chances of success increase if you become aroused through G-spot stimulation rather than clitoral stimulation, which—although less frequent—can also have the same effect. Once you have stimulated your G-spot you can also, if you want, increase your arousal with repeated penetrations from your partner. Remember that in sex all is fair if you both agree.

The amount of fluid ejaculated varies from one woman to another. It is also conditioned by multiple factors: the phase of the menstrual cycle, the degree of G-spot stimulation, the type of feelings you have toward your partner, the strength of the pelvic muscles, the kind of orgasm you are having…

Would you like to give your partner a love massage? Use the ridge that encircles your glans to reach the G-spot of the woman you are making love to. Do it slowly at first, stimulating the zone to the maximum, and don't speed up until you realize that both of you are about to ignite with pleasure. You will both reach an unforgettable orgasm.

Choose the moment of the cycle in which it's easier to ejaculate in order to try your first experiences.

- **Before menstruation.** Generally, it's easier to ejaculate during the twelve days prior to and during menstruation. And it's harder to ejaculate if you just had your period, so you should wait a few days.

- **Menopause.** If you are approaching menopause, but your period continues to be more or less regular, use the previous criteria. If, on the contrary, your period is already irregular, then any time is a good time to try it, but don't worry if you can't get it on the first try. If you have already passed menopause, you can try it out whenever you want; any time is suitable. Remember that ejaculation does not stop with your period; you can always enjoy it.

- **Pregnancy.** If you are pregnant, ejaculation could be easier than usual and it is by no means contraindicated or dangerous.

- **Contraceptives.** It is not clear whether taking contraceptives affects ejaculation or not, so women who are taking them should restrict themselves to following the recommendation regarding the twelve days prior to menstruation. If you use a diaphragm, you should know that the pressure it exerts on the urethral canal could block ejaculation flow toward the exterior and it would be advisable that you take it out beforehand.

Patience, perseverance, intimacy, and relaxation. Before we keep talking about ejaculation, prepare yourself to enjoy it. In order to do so I suggest the following steps.

- **Patience.** Each time you experiment with new techniques you must have patience; you will not always see results on the first attempt. Do you remember the first time you made love? You probably didn't reach orgasm that time and it was no reason for you to believe you were never going to enjoy sex. It's the same with ejaculation. Allow yourself the required time, appreciate every moment, and relax.

- **Perseverance.** After patience, perseverance is the attitude that will help you ejaculate. The more often you try it the easier it will be to achieve. Don't let yourself be discouraged by the first failures. After every attempt your awareness of the existence of your G-spot will increase and you will discover, additionally, new sources of pleasure.

- **Intimacy.** Make sure that you are in the proper atmosphere to relax and get carried away. That is why I suggest you try it by yourself at first. When you know how you feel, it will be easier to share it.

- **Relaxation.** Eliminate all your tension. Relax your body and get it ready to experience pleasure. Learning how to relax during erotic stimulation requires you to abandon those attitudes that tend to get the body tensed, and have a better circulation of energy. To do so, breathing is the core of all sensations and prolongs the erotic energy around your body.

Once you have gotten these preliminaries under control, you should create a pleasant space personalized for the occasion. If you have enough time, it's worth it to take a relaxing bath.

Lay out a few towels on the floor and place them so you can rest your back against the wall, a cushion, or a chair. Get a big mirror to leave in front of you. If you would like and if it relaxes you, you can also light a few sandalwood candles.

Now that you have everything ready, read the explanations I have given you to locate your G-spot again. Remember the steps you followed, how it swelled, and the pleasurable sensations you experienced. Now get ready to stimulate it. Remember, we are going to experiment with physical arousal and try to separate it from the mental one, which produces the orgasm: we are going to ejaculate without orgasm.

EJACULATE WITHOUT HAVING AN ORGASM

A guaranteed way to ejaculate is, as we have said, manual G-spot stimulation. However, not only can you ejaculate during orgasm, but you can also do it independently. It may seem less erotic, but it's good to experiment with ejaculation and to confirm you can do it. Besides, if you control it by yourself, it will also be easier to do it with your partner. I encourage you to try it, especially if you are one of those who believe you don't ejaculate. If you are aware of these sensations, you will be able to create an accurate mental image of your sexual needs, so later you can share them with your partner.

- **First phase.** Caress and stimulate your G-spot: increase stimulation until you get to a level of arousal where you

> Why do some women ejaculate and others don't? According to many specialists, if the zone is correctly simulated the liquid is surely secreted; it's just that in many cases it can be reabsorbed by the bladder, so it doesn't come out. That is why they believe they don't ejaculate.

feel you are progressively getting closer to orgasm. Check that your vagina also swells toward the exterior and that the G-spot swells visibly. The edges of the G-spot, subtle and almost imperceptible at the beginning, are growing... Can you feel it? How do you like the experience?

- **Second phase.** Pay attention to the "rise" of ejaculation. When stimulating your G-spot you will feel the urge to urinate, but this is a normal response. Another sensation that warns you that ejaculation is coming is that you will feel the pleasure go down to your feet. Slight at the beginning, these waves of pleasure will be increasingly stronger. The best way to feel and even increase them is to let them come naturally. Relax and take advantage of these moments of arousal; stop right when the heat is building and continue the stimulation later.

- **Third phase.** Keep your finger in the interior of the vagina. Stimulate your G-spot while lifting your buttocks and letting them rest on your heels. Stimulate your G-spot and contract and relax your PC muscles as if you had the urge to urinate. Stay there for a few seconds, and then go back to stimulating your G-spot. Repeat this exercise many times, without removing your finger from the vagina. You will notice that your G-spot continues to swell.

- **Fourth phase.** Keep on stimulating until the point where you are so turned on that you only want one thing—for him to penetrate you without stopping!—and you feel you have to revert to your usual technique to reach orgasm.

- **Fifth phase.** Remove your finger. Notice how you feel the urge to urinate once again. Now it's definitely the ejaculate.

- **Sixth phase.** If you want you can try it again. The female body is capable of it, so be willing to ejaculate for the second time.

> Awakening your ability to ejaculate and penetrating the mysteries of vaginal orgasms opens new doors in the discovery of a woman's sexual enjoyment and produces extremely pleasurable sensations that you will not want to miss out on again.

Treat yourself to one of the greatest pleasures: masturbation

You will have observed that, so far, in order to locate the G-spot and reach ejaculation we have been talking about self-stimulation, that is, masturbation. In fact, it's one of the most pleasurable ways of reaching orgasm, either alone or with company. Would you like to learn a few tricks to enjoy your body to the maximum? In this chapter we will examine them in detail.

Getting on the path to sexual pleasure, the orgasm is not something immediate. Men as well as women learn their own path toward the pleasure through study and practice, and often it's masturbation that offers the first clues to follow.

Masturbation, far from being something dirty or obscene (as it has been endlessly condemned in Western culture), is a pleasurable activity, natural, fun, healthy, and highly recommended for both sexes. It is totally untrue that practicing masturbation—whether done daily, less frequently, or more often—produces physical or mental illnesses. Nor is it solely a habit of immature people or adolescents. On the contrary, masturbation has its place in a healthy, adult sex life and can be done while single or in a relationship. Not to mention that with its practice it's easier to reach orgasm and that it's the simplest form of safe sex, carrying no risk of sexually transmitted diseases.

Although it's not part of our culture to encourage women to become familiar with their body and enjoy it (neither physically nor emotionally), I suggest you try it out and masturbate without prejudice. If you decide to play with your body, to get to know those corners that provide you with pleasure, you will notice yourself approaching life differently. It is a good way to become familiar with our own emotions and reactions to pleasure, and—why not?—an unbeatable way to start the day.

A study done in 1953 by renowned specialist Kinsey confirmed that 94% of women were able to reach orgasm, and 95% of those women could do so by masturbating, that is, by themselves! Haven't you ever felt like making love but your partner wasn't home? Or perhaps he didn't want to have sex at that moment? Yes? Well, if you ever need to satiate your sexual appetite, it's perfectly healthy and recommendable to do it without your partner or even while he watches you. Besides, if you masturbate together it also reduces stress caused by the idea that the only way to reach orgasm is through penetration. When masturbating women get to know their body and exactly what they like, and thus they can improve their relations with a partner because they are able to guide their partner more accurately.

The frequency of masturbation for women is variable and doesn't depend so much on whether they have relations with a partner, but more on the sexual desire they feel at any given moment. If you feel like playing, if you feel the tingling of your body asking for sexual stimulation, forget the taboos and explore what gives you the greatest pleasure. Whether in the shower, lying in bed, on the couch while watching a pornographic movie, or aided by sex toys such as vibrators, pillows, or fruits, play with your fingers and find the pleasure you are waiting for.

There is no one technique in order to stimulate oneself, but rather it depends on each woman. Some prefer to lie still, using one hand for the genitalia and the other to caress the rest of the body,

Culturally, female masturbation has been a more taboo topic than male masturbation. It's a subject that isn't usually discussed with friends or a partner. Despite this taboo, according to different studies, between 70% and 82% of women have masturbated to the point of orgasm at least once in their life. Some even begin in their twenties or after having had sexual relations with a partner.

while others move vigorously and caress their breasts and genitalia with their hands, also rubbing themselves with pillows or the sheets to increase pleasure. On other occasions, they use lubricants to more easily insert fingers into the vagina, or get help from sex toys.

If you are masturbating for the first time, try all the different techniques and objects you have access to; only after trying them all will you know which is the best one for you. Creating a good atmosphere will also help you get started. Imagine a scenario that turns you on and put on some music, surround yourself with perfume, warm light, and candles, and have a nice glass of wine or champagne. Or you might prefer something stronger and more visual, like watching a porn movie or getting help online to stimulate yourself. Don't rush, take all the time you need, and enjoy. Remember: if you can control your arousal you will also increase the intensity of your orgasm. Later, when having sex with your partner, you can experience together what you have practiced on your own.

> Doctor Niels Lauerson tells us in his book *It's Your Body*: "Learn to recognize an orgasm whenever you have one... The more these orgasms become a reflexive act, the easier it is to have them." Indeed, numerous studies also reveal that women who masturbate have orgasms three times more easily with their partner than those who never masturbate."

MEN CAN ALSO "MASTURBATE US"

When the moment is right, your partner can also use a few little tricks to "masturbate you" in order to increase your pleasure…and his. It is highly erotic to watch each other masturbating; you both will see how you get aroused with just the simple visual, and you'll discover what techniques the other enjoys the most (very valuable information).

It's best if you give him a few rough ideas, drawing up a little guide with your hand to teach him what you want him to do. Try not to let him focus only on the genitalia; your body has other parts just as "interesting" and stimulating, such as the breasts and belly button. Let him caress the clitoris, change the pace, and press on it slightly, let him see how your labia increase in size and how you squirm with pleasure. Remember at all times to maintain proper hygiene, not just on your hands, but your entire body.

IDEAS FOR MORE PLEASURABLE MASTURBATION

Although masturbating is something intimate and we are the ones who know our body and its mechanisms of pleasure best, it never hurts to learn a few little tricks for improvement.

- Start by stretching out in bed and spreading your legs wide open. Softly tap and rub your genital area; you will notice how your heart rate increases. Now you can already guess where this is going! As your arousal continues to grow from caressing the genitalia, move on to rhythmically caress your clitoris with one hand. Meanwhile, with the other hand you can stimulate another erogenous zone such as your breasts, focus on your nipples, wet your fingers with saliva, and resume massaging... your heart rate will progressively increase and you will begin to feel greater pleasure, which in turn will encourage you to keep on pressing and insert your fingers in your vagina with more desire each time. Move your fingers in a circular motion over the upper part of your clitoris. You can also stimulate and rub the area surrounding your clitoris or pull your labia back so there is more tension in the area. Rub and lightly hit it; you will soon end up having an orgasm.

The clitoris is one of the most pleasurable spots for women. Its stimulation provokes orgasm in almost all of us. Find your preferred form of stimulation. You can make a circular motion or give soft little taps with your fingers. Some women prefer direct stimulation, while others prefer lateral caresses. Explore the folds of your vagina, paying attention to the sensitivity of the labia minora, and investigate other erogenous spots, such as your breasts, belly...

- Another pleasurable option involves closing your legs tight together, on your back. Next, with one hand, softly stretch your genitalia upward and stimulate your clitoris with the other. Begin with a circular movement, very slowly and gently at first and then, as arousal increases, move more vigorously, according to what your body demands from you. Slow down if you want to control your arousal and speed up again until finishing with a more pleasurable and controlled orgasm.

• With sheets, pajamas, or underwear make a ball the size of a fist. Lie facedown, with the ball under your clitoris. Move your hips in circles over it. If you continue this massage for some time, while caressing your breasts or other parts of your body, you will end up reaching orgasm.

• Begin stretched out on your back and use any of the previous techniques to reach a certain degree of arousal and lubrication of your vagina, but without letting yourself approach orgasm. Then, with your legs open and relaxed, insert a finger and move it in and out of your vagina; you can also add a circular movement to this one, as if you were screwing something. Meanwhile, if you want, you can stimulate your clitoris or breasts with the other hand. Another technique involves placing your palm over your clitoris, using only one hand, and inserting your fingers in the vagina, softly massaging it. You can increase the number of fingers and change the intensity of the massage, depending on how you like it.

• Laying face up, insert a finger in your vagina just as we have indicated in the previous techniques, and place your thumb over your clitoris to caress it. With the other hand you can massage your breasts. Push your body up and down, aided by your feet, along with the insertion of your finger and the clitoral stimulation. At first keep your legs spread but when you feel the orgasm coming, close them and feel the muscle contractions.

• Begin by stimulating the pubic area with any of the previous techniques. Once you are aroused, place your other hand by the anus. First touch it with circular movements or up and down. Then, without rushing, try inserting one finger inside. Perhaps at the beginning you struggle a little; it's difficult to get into without lubrication, either with objects or our own fingers, but you will see the satisfaction you can reach with proper stimulation. In order to facilitate the insertion of your fingers, lubricate them with some Vaseline.

- You can also masturbate by rubbing your thighs together. Rhythmically rub, applying a light pressure on your clitoris. Pressure leads little by little to climax. You can do this naked or clothed, in bed or seated.

- If you share your house with other people you might consider it difficult to masturbate; however, it shouldn't be a problem because you can take advantage of the privacy that the bathroom provides. Besides the previous techniques, you can practice new ones or combine those. If you decide to use the bathroom, lie down in the bathtub and direct the shower stream over your vagina, mons pubis, and clitoris. Change the water pressure and temperature. It's best to use a steady stream of slightly warm water for greater stimulation. Open your labia and expose your clitoris to the stream of water. You can move your hips to prolong the pleasure, while you increase the water pressure as you feel your arousal increase.

It's not always possible to reach orgasm. You may not have reached orgasm after practicing all the techniques I've proposed to you. Don't worry, there is surely an explanation and, as soon as you overcome the issue, you will be able to enjoy your body to the maximum:

- Maybe you have tried these exercises on a day you have been too tense or too alert worrying about people coming into your room. Try to ignore these circumstances or find a time when you can avoid these concerns.

- Did it hurt when inserting your fingers in your vagina? You might not be lubricated enough; if your vaginal fluid is not enough, try it with your own saliva or use lubricants.

- Are you focusing too much on the goal of orgasming? Sometimes, when we are over-anticipating the outcome, it's more likely that we fail. Go with the flow and don't worry about the moment you will reach orgasm, it will come on its own.

- You are too relaxed and that doesn't "turn you on." Not all of us react or stimulate ourselves in the same way. Maybe you are one of those who needs to perform near a window, thinking that somebody will enjoy the scene, or maybe you prefer wearing sexy underwear. Try it, don't feel shy. Everything you try in order to reach pleasure, without harming others, is allowed.

- If you have your period it may be harder for you to reach orgasm than it is at a different stage of your cycle. I suggest you try it between the tenth and eighteenth day of your cycle, when your hormone levels are higher.

Other erogenous spots: the A-, K-, and U-spots

As we have said, there are other spots located in our genitalia that are also highly erogenous zones, though the G-spot is the one that helps us reach the most satisfying orgasms and leads to ejaculation. In this chapter we are going to highlight the other erogenous spots—their location, their most effective direct stimulation, and the sexual positions that are the most satisfying.

I advise you to read this chapter with your partner, because he can benefit a lot from the knowledge of these "secret" zones in women.

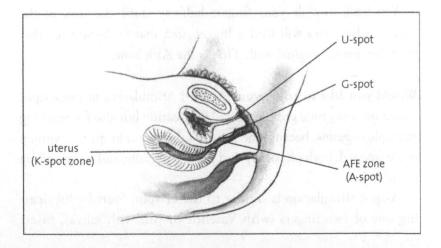

THE A-SPOT

The A-spot, or AFE (Anterior Fornix Erotic zone) spot, was discovered in 1996. During research carried out by Asian scientists on vaginal dryness, it was discovered that 95% of women become aroused by stimulating this zone. Indeed, many of them got to have their first orgasm or more intense orgasms than previously experienced. Studies done later concluded that out of the 193 women whose A-spot was stimulated, 182 experienced very intense pleasure.

REMEMBER
Stimulation of the A-spot produces:
- Greater, faster, and longer lubrication
- Greater arousal
- Multiple orgasms

Do you want to find it? This spot is located in the front part of the vagina (see the diagram on the previous page), about ¾ or 1 inch before the cervix, a little deeper than the G-spot. Its surface is soft and very sensitive to touch: a small mass of spongy tissue.

You have to slide your fingers halfway along the wall of the vagina, where you will find a bigger area that is slightly rougher than the normal vaginal wall. That is the AFE zone.

Would you like to enjoy your A-spot? Stimulation of the A-spot allows not only for a greater vaginal lubrication but also for reaching multiple orgasms, because the greater lubrication keeps the woman more aroused, both physically and psychologically, and more willing to enjoy it.

A-spot stimulation is similar to the G-spot. Start by lubricating one or two fingers (with Vaseline or just with saliva), insert them into your vagina, and look for the A-spot. In order to stimulate it manually you need to keep your fingers straight and make a swinging movement around it. Be aware that your fingers are not the only means of A-spot stimulation; you can also do it during coitus, in positions where his penis hits the anterior part of your vagina:

- **Dragonfly position.** Both partners lie on their sides, in a comfortable place such as the bed. She has her back to him, one body molded into the other. Displaying her skill, she flexes her upper leg and opens the door of pleasure; the man penetrates her by leveraging himself using her leg, which is rested on his hips. The sexy things he can whisper into her ear are the perfect spice to get maximum pleasure. Penetration goes halfway in, so the pleasure comes from the desire for it to go gradually deeper and trigger the most amazing orgasm.

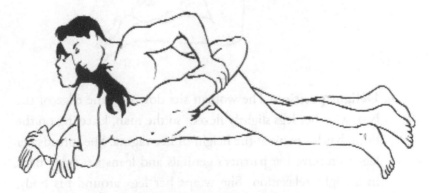

- **Wild Furor position.** Also known as "doggy style," it is the one that many animals use. It is a form of passionate and wild coitus. She gets down on her hands and knees, while he penetrates her from behind. It's a comfortable position, particularly for men, who can touch their partner's breasts or clitoris.

The woman, in turn, can caress his testicles. This position is also very common for anal coitus. The *Kamasutra* tells us about this posture: "In the ardor of copulation, a pair of lovers becomes blind with passion and continues with great impetuosity, without any thought of excess."

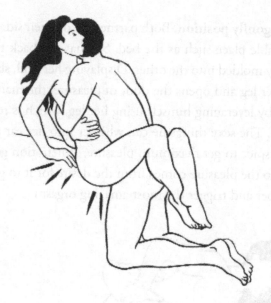

- **Delight position.** The woman sits down on the edge of the bed, with her legs slightly flexed, so the man, kneeling on the floor, has his penis at the height of her vagina. She spreads her legs to receive her partner's genitals and leans her body back in a slight relaxation. She wraps her legs around his body, while he takes charge of the pace of penetration.

THE K-SPOT

The K-spot was discovered in 1998 by an American, Barbara Keesling, and she named it "the mysterious passage" since it remained hidden for so long. With the results of her studies, Keesling published a book titled *Super Sexual Orgasm*. The reason for its secrecy is that it is located at the final part of the vagina, just before the cervix, making it hard to access.

The K-spot is hidden due to pressure of the uterus, so in the majority of cases it is inaccessible in sexual relations unless you are aware of its existence. Its stimulation leads to extremely intense orgasms through the whole vagina from the innermost part outward; it is called a "big top orgasm."

Would you like to enjoy your K-spot? It is possible to stimulate it during coitus with a position in which the penis goes deeply inside the vagina. The man faces the woman, who lies face up and places her legs on his shoulders. A word of advice: penetration is even deeper and more pleasurable if she is at the edge of the bed and he is kneeling on the floor, so her vagina is at the height of his penis.

The weight and position of the uterus compresses the vagina at the top where the K-spot is located, impeding its stimulation. By performing the PC muscle exercises, it's possible, among other benefits, to elevate the uterus, thus stimulating the K-spot and achieving tremendous orgasms.

THE U-SPOT OR URETHRAL SPOT

The U-spot (or urethral spot) was discovered by Kevin McKenna. It is an area very close to the urethra (the place where women pass urine) that is located underneath the clitoris. Just like the clitoris, the urethra is also a pleasurable spot for some women, which is logical if we keep in mind that the urethra (with its paraurethral glands) is surrounded by the clitoris on three sides and located between the glans of the clitoris and the vaginal entrance (introitus). The urethra, where the female body discharges urine, is just below the clitoris and above the vagina. Remember that the clitoris is much bigger than it seems to be, which indicates how arousing it could stimulate the urethra.

Do you want to enjoy your U-spot? It is very easy to stimulate the U-spot manually. Some women claim that they like to firmly press on their urethral zone when they masturbate to increase their pleasure. Since this zone is pretty small, in order to concentrate sensation in the proper place you should begin by making soft circular caresses or moving your fingers up and down, pressing a little.

For good oral stimulation you should spread your labia minora so the urethral zone is totally exposed. It can be stimulated by tongue movements. To get more pressure he can also use his chin or lower lip, pushing with his teeth. In fact, coital stimulation, by penetration, is not the best method for U-spot stimulation: oral is better. However some positions favor its arousal:

- **The woman on top and leaning forward.** Her legs should be spread wide open, so that penetration is deep and allows contact between the base of the penis and the urethral zone. You can also sit on a low chair or cushion and wrap your legs around your man (he should kneel down in front of you). This type of orgasm with the woman on top is possible if the woman leans forward a lot, with her legs open to get the maximum contact of the vaginal entrance with the base of her partner's penis.

- **Standing or kneeling.** You can also stimulate the U-spot by having sex standing, seated, or kneeling. In order to do so, the man should give short thrusts while she wraps her legs around him. Again, the position in which she is seated on the bed's edge and he is kneeling on the floor is good for stimulating this area.

Arousal of this zone is very pleasurable, but orgasms are rare if only the U-spot is stimulated, even though it's full of nerve endings.

ORAL TECHNIQUES FOR U-SPOT ORGASM

One of the most common techniques is the one in which the man presses firmly and steadily on the urethral zone with his lower lip and teeth while performing oral sex (being extremely careful to avoid hurting her). Also, it's good to separate the labia minora so the urethral zone is totally exposed and to softly caress it with your tongue. Her reaction will immediately indicate if she likes it and you should continue down that road.

LET'S SUM IT UP

- In the interior of the vagina there is a zone that is extremely sensitive to firm pressure. It is located at the anterior wall of the vagina, about two inches from the entrance, and it is called the "G-spot."

- Every woman has this spot.

- When it receives proper stimulation, the G-spot dilates and produces an orgasm.

- At the moment of orgasm, many women ejaculate through the urethra a liquid similar to the male ejaculate, though it doesn't contain sperm.

- As a consequence of G-spot stimulation a woman may experience multiple orgasms.

- For some women it's difficult to stimulate the G-spot properly if she is lying stretched out. Other positions provide more pleasurable sensations.

- The liquid produced during female ejaculation should not be confused with urine.

- The strength that a woman is able to exert with her pubococcygeus muscle is directly related to the ability to reach orgasm during intercourse.

- Women can do the simple Kegel's exercises to train their pubococcygeus muscles.

- There are different types of orgasms for women. The vulvar orgasm (triggered by the clitoris), the uterine orgasm (experienced right after intercourse), and the mixed orgasm.

Whole body source of pleasure

The erogenous zones are those parts of our body where caresses produce more pleasurable sensations. They are zones that concentrate high quantities of nerve endings, making them respond with an extra sensitivity to stimulation. One of the most interesting adventures we can engage in with our partner is, precisely, to stimulate each of these erotic spots with caresses and massages. This increases the initial erotic charge, because touch is the first form of contact with the other and a way to see our partner's reactions. There is a wide range of caresses that will awaken the senses for both of you until reaching climax. This practice offers infinite variations and incomparable moments of passion.

The search for our partner's erogenous zones can begin at any part of the body, from the feet all the way up to the eyelids, including arms, thighs, nape of the neck, hair… It will just be a simple starting point, because the entire body is waiting to be explored and stimulated. It is preferable to begin first in the most highly erogenous zones and then move over to the rest of the body.

Remember it's not good to always repeat the same caresses, in the same manner, in the same places. Mechanical repetition can cause a feeling of rejection and even make your partner unwilling to continue with the sexual act.

There are two different types of erogenous zones in the human body:

- **The primary zones** are those parts of the body considered more erogenous because they respond better to any sensual touch and they are the best way to get the partner aroused. Stimulating those zones is a direct invitation to have sex. If you are a man you can start by caressing her nipples or clitoris, and if you are a woman you can start with his penis or testicles.

- **The secondary zones**, such as the neck, center of the back, ears, throat, lips, front part of the legs, or anus, are parts of the body that respond with high levels of pleasure and arousal, though less intense than the primary zones. Don't forget about them in your most erotic moments.

Skin on skin contact is one of the major components of sexual activity, thus it's important to learn to caress yourself and to allow others to caress you. There is no need to focus on the common erogenous zones alone, because skin is made up of infinite sensitive spots that can be discovered every day. Remember: the entire body is an enormous erogenous zone, though in some spots sensations are more intense than in others.

Since each person has an exclusive erogenous map, it's important for each of us to explore our own bodies and to discover our most erogenous parts. Not every stimulation of a particular erogenous zone will always be pleasurable; it depends on many factors, from the skill of the lover to the predisposition of the receiver.

LOVING FOREPLAY

Foreplay is critically important to the sexual encounter because it prepares the body for sex and makes it more satisfying.

It is important to regard these affectionate gestures with the importance they deserve because they allow us to feel sexier, trust our partner, and enjoy a more complete sexual encounter. Never forget that sexual relations are not just coitus and orgasm, but a wide range of games, caresses, hugs, affectionate words, oral exploration, and massages that make the sexual organs become organs of pleasure. It has been proven that women need foreplay more than men to enjoy coitus and to reach orgasm. The simple act of undressing a woman can be so charged with eroticism and sensuality that it can be used as a warm-up game before coitus, looking for new innovations in every encounter. Every detail, every little insinuation increases desire in the couple, and the great secret is about alternating the sexual games to always keep things spicy, thus avoiding the sensation of falling into a mere routine.

Have you ever tried putting his condom on? A very sensual and acrobatic way of doing it is with your mouth, and it is one of the sexiest games...

The importance of games and foreplay. During foreplay the skin, and more precisely, the erogenous zones are stimulated. These zones change from one person to another, but the most common are the mouth, ears, nape of the neck, buttocks, belly, inner thighs, feet, nipples, clitoris, vulva, and vagina (particularly the G-spot) for women, and the scrotum and nipples for men. The genital zones are particularly sensitive to stimulation for both sexes, so they must be treated with special care.

Foreplay is of great importance in sexual relations, because it prepares the body for coitus and orgasm. Sexual arousal is induced by a complex mixture of mental and physical exercises. Contrary to common belief, men also need foreplay that provides the required stimulation to get a firm erection (though if he suffers premature ejaculation it can be reduced to the minimum). In the case of women, this stage is especially important, because for a woman to be fully aroused her body often needs extended stimulation. This foreplay makes the vagina dilate and start lubricating, which facilitates penetration and provides the necessary degree of arousal to be able to reach orgasm.

Creating a suitable atmosphere is always useful for practicing foreplay. Put on sensual music and dim natural light; serve two glasses of fine wine and light incense. You can start dressed and then mutually undress each other. The simple visual stimulation from watching her undoing her bra or him unzipping his pants can elevate the temperature in the room up to uncontainable levels of desire.

Now let's take a closer look at these erogenous zones:

HAIR

Massaging the scalp produces a very pleasant relaxation, so it is advised both at the beginning and end of the sexual act. Use your thumbs to softly massage in circles, especially on the temples and the middle of the forehead. On the other hand, hair also works to provide pleasure and many men get aroused when their partner brushes his back with her hair.

EYES

Eyelids are full of nerve endings, so kissing, softly licking, and caressing them with fingers produces very nice and stimulating sensations.

EARS

Ears are very sensitive parts of the body (particularly the back and earlobe) and, contrary to common belief, men's ears are more sensitive than women's. Try this technique and you will see the results you stir up. Insert the tip of your tongue inside his ear and trace little circles. Then, lick his earlobe and press it between your lips, softly tightening. You can repeat those moves and alternate with caresses in other areas. You can also blow a little by the back of the ear. Add a dose of soft whispers to these caresses and he will surely melt with pleasure.

MOUTH

Sensitivity of the lips increases with arousal, making them sensitive to the touch and caress of other lips. The tongue can give soft caresses on any part of your partner's body and, to many people, it's the most sensual and arousing sexual game.

NECK, NAPE, AND SHOULDERS

With your hands or mouth it's possible to stimulate these especially sensitive zones and produce pleasurable tingles. If your partner is a man, proceed energetically because the skin of his neck is thicker and many men get aroused with an aggressive mouth. If your partner is a woman, kiss, lick, and caress her neck, and softly massage her shoulders. Psychologically, the nape transmits feelings of trust to the one who receives the caress and affection to the one who carries it out.

CHEST

A man's chest responds sexually to stimulation, although it's less sensitive than a woman's. Chests can be stimulated in multiple ways: caressing, massaging, kissing, licking, etc. Try this: cover his chest with wet kisses, from top to bottom, and give him little licks; then, blow on the wet surface. This switch between cold and warm turns out to be very arousing. Masturbating the man with his penis in between her breasts is a really sexy practice, pressing her breasts together so his penis is held firmly and making vertical movements simulating coitus. On the other hand, a woman's nipples are extremely sensitive and he can blow, suck, pinch, and press them in between his lips while giving subtle licks with his tongue.

ARMS

A soft manual stimulation over the armpit area and the inner part of the forearm can be very pleasurable if you avoid tickling. The inner part of the elbow is a very erogenous secondary zone, so it's useful to combine it with other zones. And regarding the hands, they have more than 40,000 nerve endings waiting to be stimulated. Place your partner's hand over your mouth and go over the palm with only the tip of the tongue; it's an unusual and very arousing sensation. Another technique is to trace circles with your fingers from the inside to the outside (in a spiral) of your partner's palm. Go up and down his fingers with just the tips of yours, and caress them softly. The nervous receptivity of fingers is normally used to sense textures and the shape of objects, and this sensitivity becomes a very suitable way to feel your partner's body.

BACK

Caressing your partner from the shoulders to the base of the spine while your partner lies facedown can be much more erotic than if you are watching each other. Along both sides of the spine is a set of nerves that can be stimulated very effectively, either manually or orally, and either ascending or descending. In front of the sacrum, where back and butt join together, there is an area more sensitive than the rest. It would be more pleasurable if you start by the neck and go down progressively following the spine, stopping with soft massages. My advice is that you sit on your partner's butt so you both can feel the other's skin.

BELLY

The belly responds very well to soft rubs and kisses. The area around the belly button is very sensitive in women, while in men it is the zone that goes from the belly button to the pubis that is full of nerve endings. In order to arouse them, trace a vertical line with your tongue and lips. Lick, suck, bite. You can trace a horizontal line across the abdomen, from hip to hip.

GROIN

It is especially sensitive for men. Go over it with your fingers and give a soft massage from the hips to the deep muscle. Combine it with kisses on the inner thighs and caress them with your fingers toward his penis, up to the base of his testicles. Press the perineum a few times. This technique can be an excellent prologue to oral sex.

THIGHS

The inner part of the thigh, where the skin is softer, is a very sensitive area that can be a source of pleasure if it is caressed, licked, or kissed. Try rubbing in circles or sliding your hands upward over the back part of the leg.

BUTTOCKS

They contain a lot of nerve endings that can be stimulated by little spanks or by rubbing. On women, massages that lift and open them work better than the ones that push and close them. If your partner is a man, once aroused, you can drive him crazy with passion by spanking, pinching, or massaging his butt. If you make love in the missionary position, don't miss the chance to softly spank or squeeze his buttocks.

PROSTATE

It is the so-called male G-spot because of the intense sensations it produces. The only way to reach this muscle directly is through the anus, though it can also be stimulated through the perineum.

ANUS

Highly sensitive for both sexes, it can be best stimulated with soft circular movements with a fingertip or with the tip of the tongue.

PERINEUM

The area between the genital organs and the anus is very sensitive to stimulation, though not too many people know how to benefit from it. For women, this zone reacts very well to pressure with fingers or to circular caresses, and for men, it's even more sensitive because the prostate is right underneath the skin. Press firmly with one or two fingers on the skin located below the scrotum, for no more than a second. Repeat various times. Oral sex in combination with perineum stimulation can be extremely pleasurable.

FEET

Feet are full of nerve endings. Coat your hands with oil before touching them to better slide in between the toes. Whatever you do with the feet, try not to tickle them. You can begin with soft massages on the soles, starting by the ankles and going down all the way to the toes, stretching and massaging each one of them. Finish up with a massage on the bridge of the feet. Besides massaging, you might dare to play a more sensual game, such as sucking, licking, little bites, etc. Using your feet to play with your partner's genitals can be a very satisfying sexual game. Of course, it's important to be very careful, because there is not as much control with feet as there is with hands, and we can hurt our partner.

Our
Kamasutra

In the two previous chapters you have learned to enjoy your body thoroughly; you even know about your most remote zones. You know how to orgasm by masturbating and how to ejaculate. And you also know that arousal reached by sharing sexual games with your partner can provide very intense pleasures, because the sensations implicit in the union of two individuals is something unrivaled.

REMEMBER

Women have two main points of arousal: the clitoris and the G-spot. And men also have two major arousal spots: the penis and the prostate gland. The clitoris, located on the exterior of the body, next to the entrance of the vagina, is easy to discover and to have fun stimulating. The G-spot, located on the front wall of the vagina, is harder to find, but can make you enjoy multiple orgasms or more intense orgasms, especially if it is your partner who stimulates it. For men, the penis is also easy to stimulate, while the prostate, accessed through the anterior wall of the rectum, can be complicated without the help of another person.

In this chapter we propose a set of sex positions that will drive you both to ecstasy. If you have a long-term partner, you already know that routine is the worst enemy of sexual relations and, in order to get rid of it, couples practice numerous positions when making love. Do you dare stop proceeding with "business as usual"? Would you like to learn positions that can lead you to orgasms you only dared to dream of? If, on the other hand, you have sporadic partners, what could be better than giving your one-night stand a legendary memory of the night you met each other? Be willing to discover new sensations and to enjoy them with company.

MISSIONARY

This is one of the most universal positions, not that it's precisely boring. Additionally, many associate it with love and romance, the beginning of the couple, or adolescence, but it's worth experiencing it at every stage of your sexual life and to get the most from it. Being face to face allows for infinite variants, making it more attractive and arousing. Mobility of the hands, proximity of the faces, and comfort for the bodies are its main advantages, although it's also ideal for trying new caresses during coitus: she could touch the buttocks and anus of her partner; he could rub her clitoris or she could do it herself, the legs of both could be closer together to feel some struggle during penetration.

There is a variant of this posture that takes pleasurable sensations to the extreme. The woman remains lying face up with her legs spread and flexed, resting her arms behind her shoulders near the nape of her neck. When her partner is ready to penetrate her, she lifts her hips and supports herself on her partner's folded legs. The pleasure she receives comes from deep penetration, the possibility of touching the G-spot, and the feeling of the whole vaginal and abdominal zone, wrapped up in the man's body. The fatigue you

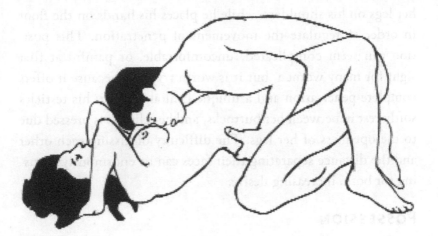

will experience trying to hold this position is rewarded with the powerful orgasm you can achieve.

THE COWGIRL

In this position the woman is on top, which is really arousing for many men who are used to the missionary position. This way she can rub her clitoris against his belly more easily, setting her own rhythm. It is ideal for women who have trouble reaching orgasm and need a more direct stimulation of the clitoris and labia, because he can stimulate them with his hands. Additionally, he can take the opportunity to caress her buttocks, insert a finger in her anus, and pull her toward him by grabbing her butt.

TAKE THE PLUNGE

This is a position of total penetration that leads to the most intense orgasms. With her back on the floor, she waits for her partner to introduce his penis into her vagina; then she rests her legs on his shoulders, while he places his hands on the floor in order to regulate the movement of penetration. This position can seem complicated, uncomfortable, or painful at first sight for many women, but it is worth trying it because it offers complete penetration and a unique genital contact: his testicles softly rest in between her buttocks, and her clitoris is pressed due to the openness of her legs. The difficulty of kissing each other and the distance separating their faces can be enormously arousing for both, increasing desire.

POSSESSION

Both partners intertwine their legs in this sensual and pleasurable position. The woman remains lying with her legs apart waiting for her partner, who is seated, to penetrate her. Then, by grabbing her by her shoulders, he regulates the movement and cadence of penetration. His penis goes in and out, deviating its movement downward, because the woman's belly is slightly higher than his. If you have paid attention to the explanation for G-spot

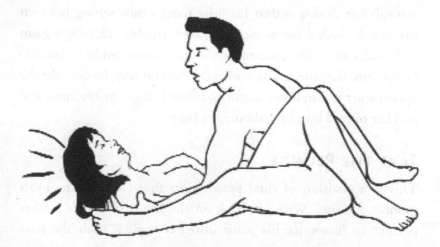

stimulation you will see how this position makes it easier for his penis to reach that zone.

CLIMBING THE TREE

Sometimes we can't wait to get to the bed for making love because the desire is so intense that it demands a quick satisfaction of our sexual needs. This is what could happen if you try this position. He is standing up, naked and facing her, very aroused after an ardent foreplay. She climbs her partner and embraces him with her legs while wrapping her arms around his neck, initiating some sensual kisses. He holds her by her buttocks and pulls her toward him for penetration. "Climbing the tree" is a passionate and creative kind of sex, with complete body contact. The rhythm of coitus can have two modes: up and down, or back and forth, depending on the intensity of pleasure. It is a position for the most athletic and passionate, and it makes it possible to make love in unsuspecting places.

DELIGHT

She sits on the edge of the bed, couch, or chair, while he kneels so that his penis is at the same height as her vagina. The woman, leaning back, wraps her legs around her partner's body and relaxes to receive him and all his power, and reach orgasm. (see drawing on page 88).

THE ARMCHAIR

Supported on a pillow, the man sits with his legs flexed and partially open. This position allows her to sit comfortably in the space formed by his body. With the help of his hands, the man lowers her onto his erection, controlling both the rhythm and intensity of the penetration. Her legs rest gently on his shoulders and his head is caught between her thighs. The man can caress her clitoris as he holds her waist firmly. The difficulty of bringing your faces together and the audacity of it make this a sensual and pleasurable position.

THE SCREW

This is one of the best positions for women who have difficulty reaching orgasm through penetration, since it presses the clitoris as the vagina is penetrated, stimulating both areas at the same time. She lies on the edge of the bed and, with her back to the bed, she turns her legs to one side (each woman will know which side is more comfortable). This way the clitoris is trapped between her thighs to reach orgasm through the labia. The woman can contract and relax the whole area, while he penetrates her, kneeling in front of her and touching her breasts. Maximum pleasure guaranteed!

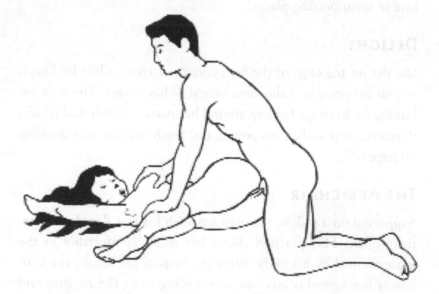

THE CATAPULT

For women, this position is an endless source of pleasure because, during coitus, it combines certain areas that other positions don't touch. She, lying face up, lifts her hips to rest them on her partner's thighs as he kneels. The woman stretches her legs and rests them on his torso or bends them to rest her feet against his chest (the second option requires less physical strength). The man has easy access to the clitoris, so he can stimulate it before beginning penetration. They both set the rhythm, depending on their desire and her flexibility.

FUSION

The man sits with his body reclined slightly back and his hands at his sides. He can stretch out or bend his legs, and his head should be relaxed. The woman assumes the active role, positioning her legs around her partner and leaning on her hands, ready to set the pace. The partners should begin with intense stimulation, since during penetration it is difficult to stimulate each other manually or orally. The woman sets the rhythm or they both move together to thrust the penis and vagina together. Either way, it is essential to take advantage of the impact to stimulate the clitoris and reach more pleasurable sensations. The gaze is also a fundamental component, and talking can also be a powerful tool to enjoy total fusion.

There is a variation of this position in which the man relaxes and lies flat out while the woman rests her feet on his shoulders and softly joins in. In this variation the penetration is deeper. She continues to set the rhythm and it's easiest to move up and down over her partner. Her hands can touch his chest or his penis before penetration, as if she were masturbating him.

THE ACROBAT

This position, not suitable for stiff bodies, may seem uncomfortable but if you are flexible enough, it can be really pleasurable. He lies down, relaxed and erect; she lets herself fall back slowly against his torso, supporting herself with her hands and initiating penetration. She bends her knees and leans back so the penis does not slip out. To activate movement, she lifts her belly, while he has easy access to her clitoris and breasts. She will end up spent from so much pleasure, making the orgasm more exciting.

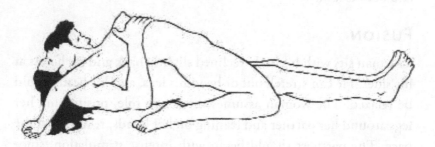

THE WHEELBARROW

The woman, at the edge of the bed and leaning on her forearms, allows herself to be "lifted" by her legs as if she were a wheelbarrow. Then the man, standing behind her, penetrates her while holding her thighs firmly. The stimulation and pleasure is centered in the genitals, but it is the man who sets the rhythm, pulling her body close to his. This position allows for a surprising array of movements and sensations: circular, up and down, with her legs more closed or open. It's easy to reach her G-spot in this position; try it and you won't regret it.

THE TRAPEZE

The man sits with his legs open and his partner positions herself on top of him, while he holds her by the wrists. She relaxes while he leans back to lie on his back. The woman should feel completely relaxed and give herself to the strength of her partner, who pulls her toward him and thrusts forcefully to reach orgasm. This is a complicated position because it requires the woman to let herself go completely, as well as a lot of balance from both partners and some strength and skill from the man. It's ideal for a change of routine and to try new sensations, but only for experienced lovers.

THE HAMMOCK

The man sits (preferably on a hard surface), with his legs bent, holding them behind the knees. The woman gets comfortable in the space between his legs and torso. He presses his knees against her body and pulls her close to him, making them both sway as he, for example, kisses or sucks on her breasts, which are level with his face.

THE WINDMILL

The woman lies face up with her legs open and lets her partner penetrate her. This position allows for a variety of sensations: the clitoris and labia are in full contact with his pelvis and the base of his penis, and penetration is best done in circular movements. The woman can caress her partner's buttocks, gently rake her nails down the back of his knees, or caress his testicles. For his part, he can lick her feet, bite her toes, caress her genitals, and penetrate her at will.

THE MOLD

With her legs together and bent (in order to press the penis), the woman lies on her side and relaxes her head back as he penetrates her, either in the vagina or the anus (this is an excellent position for anal sex). The movements should be soft and coordinated, and the penetration slow and deep: both bodies mold together like puzzle pieces. "The Mold" is ideal for women who have problems reaching orgasm or like to rub their clitoris during sex. The legs pressed together have this effect; enjoy it.

THE AMAZON

In this position, the man relaxes and lies face up with his legs slightly open and bent to his chest, waiting for the woman to squat in front of him and deliver pleasure to both of them. The woman guides her partner's penis and all the movement comes from her thighs, with the penetration going up and down. Only suitable for open minds and risk takers, "the Amazon" is the woman who rides her man wildly and primitively to an unforgettable orgasm.

THE MIRROR

She lies face up and lifts her legs. He kneels and holds her legs, one arm on the ground to keep his balance. This position allows him to vary the direction of penetration and the openness of her legs to vary the pleasure. Their faces can't approach each other and they can't do much with their hands, which generates an exciting impatience.

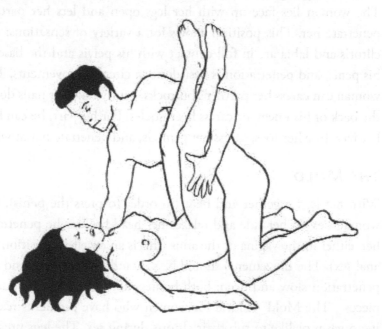

BREAKING IN

The man sits comfortably and waits to receive his partner, who mounts him, moving until reaching climax. The woman can do some foreplay and massage his penis with her hands, maintaining sexual tension without letting him penetrate her. Meanwhile, the man can look her in the eyes and impose his will, drawing her slowly onto his member. The passion and force of the embrace (culminating in explosive penetration), as well as the chance to play with their tongues and caress each other's backs, increases the excitement. This position is a direct road to orgasm, and if the penetration is done skillfully, he can reach her G-spot easily.

Another option is for the woman to position herself with her back to her partner, setting the rhythm with her feet on the ground, increasing the pleasure that comes with penetration from behind. Meanwhile, the man can caress her breasts or kiss her neck as she moves and establishes the rhythm of coitus.

THE JELLYFISH

This position is a great variation for lovers who can maintain a rocking motion during coitus that can make it more pleasurable. The man squats with his legs wide open and receives his partner, who puts her legs over his thighs to initiate a movement like a hammock, rocking forward and back with her feet firmly planted on the ground. The other option is that he stays still and lets her move. In "the Jellyfish," her chest sinks into his and they achieve a perfect connection that allows them to reach intense sensations.

Appendix:
The male G-spot

For both men and women the path to pleasure can be sinuous and strewn with obstacles. We get closer and farther from our sexual goals to end up complementing our partner at the moment of sexual enjoyment.

Finding the G-spot can mean, for many of us, something so complicated at first, like the quest for the Holy Grail, but for men theirs is also a mystery! So, the first question is the same one we had for us women: is there any key spot in men that, through its stimulation, leads to certain orgasm? The answer seems to be affirmative, though with some nuances, as we will see next.

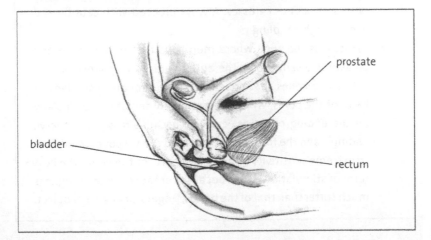

prostate

bladder

rectum

According to Dr. Jean Veláis, a specialist in male sexuality, a clever woman would realize that her partner also has an organ which, when stimulated, brings him rapidly closer to orgasm. But it's not always that easy, because not all the women caress the arousing zone, called "men's erection spot B" and located in the perineum between the scrotum and the anus. To stimulate it, a soft and firm pressure is enough, delivering so much pleasure so quickly that it can accentuate the erection and even lead directly to ejaculation. From "B-spot" to "G-spot" there is just a short step in the sex alphabet, don't you think?

Although the caress seems superficial, the prostate, which is the organ stimulated, is the actual center of male pleasure. And if "there is no analogous G-spot in men, they indeed enjoy the pressure on their prostate during anal palpation and some similarities can be drawn between the two," Dr. Jean Veláis acknowledges in his work. Additionally, the origin of its organic tissues is, curiously, the same as that of the famous female G-spot.

THE MALE GENITALS

- **TESTICLES.** They are extremely sensitive and can be stimulated with soft licks or caresses. Always proceed with caution and avoid rough handling.
- **PENIS.** It is the zone where men have the most intense and pleasurable sensations. The entire penis is very sensitive, but it has two zones that are especially erogenous: the glans or head of the penis, which are extremely sensitive, particularly on the ending part (the "crown") because it is rich in nerve endings; and the frenulum (also called the V-spot of men). Due to extreme sensitivity of these two parts of the penis, the best form of stimulation is oral, because contact from the tongue is much softer than that of the hands, fingers, or any other object.

You can give little taps with the tip of your tongue and soft licks following imaginary circles over it, then switching between vertical and horizontal licks. If you are using your fingers or any other part of the body or an object, it is important to have the area well lubricated so the contact is as gentle as possible.

THE PROSTATE, A KEY ZONE OF PLEASURE

The prostate, a small gland the size and shape of a nut located below the bladder and traversed by the urethra, takes part in sperm production, pleasure, and the ejaculation that comes after. At the moment of ejaculation and after the ejaculating canals are filled, the prostate contracts and the prostatic secretions mix with the seminal liquid. Afterward, the contraction of the bulbeocavernous muscles pushes the sperm to the urethra, and these muscular tremors are the ones that increase pleasurable sensations. When the prostate is stimulated to the point of ejaculation, the liquid often flows out softly instead of in spurts, although the amount is similar to a normal ejaculation.

The prostate is an organ of the male reproductive system that, when stimulated, causes intense orgasms. Although it doesn't seem like it, it is easy to locate and stimulate. Since the prostate is accessed through the anus, many men reject the idea because they associate it with homosexuality. However, both things have nothing to do with each other, because anal pleasure is one thing and sexual attraction for same-sex persons is another. Stimulation of the prostate is also commonly thought to be dirty and painful, which is exactly the opposite of what he will experience during this process.

Practical guide. Stimulation of the prostate via the anus is one of those practices that men appreciate more each time they try it. In order to do it, she must introduce a finger into her partner's anus to reach the gland and its borders. This practice requires a lot of delicacy (it demands a good lubrication) so the stimulation is pleasant and by no means painful.

The man must position himself with his legs folded against his chest to facilitate the entrance of the finger into his rectum (about 2 inches). The prostate can be located in this area by pressing toward the penis. Next, it should be slowly and softly massaged; the finger can press or move from the outside to the inside until reaching orgasm.

DARE TO STIMULATE HIS G-SPOT

"I like when my partner inserts her fingers in my anus, deeply, while she orally and manually stimulates my penis; it is an incomparable sensation and that's how I get the best orgasms, though other times we do it in the traditional way."

Carlos, 32 years old

If the man receives an adequate massage and stimulation of the prostate he will unavoidably reach orgasm. And his partner has the advantage; she is the only one capable of providing it, because he can't stimulate himself very easily due to its location. Do you want to try it? Remember a few rules and you will drive him crazy!

- You will be able to feel the nut-shaped prostate if you delicately insert one finger through the anal canal and direct it along its front wall.

- Once you have reached it, press in the direction of his penis until you notice a small bulge.

- The ideal position is to have him lie facing up with his knees against his chest.

- Give him a soft and slow massage until you bring him to orgasm, which will be very intense.

- The anal tissue is very easily damaged, so you need to be extremely careful and use lubricant.

- Do you want him to experience double the pleasure? Provide him with even greater pleasure by stimulating his G-spot while you perform oral sex on him or while he is penetrating you.

SUGGESTIONS

- Hygiene, always essential, is even more important for anal play.
- To avoid damaging his anus always keep your nails well cut.
- Use latex gloves or a condom to ensure greater protection and gentleness.
- Spread a water-based lubricant on your finger so penetration is easier.
- Before you introduce it, touch the external part of his anus so he relaxes and becomes receptive to this sexual practice.
- Start by introducing only a centimeter of your fingertip into the anal canal and then progressively move in circles to stimulate him.
- Continue to ask him what sensations each movement produces, and if you notice any discomfort stop immediately. Remember that sexual activities must be something pleasurable, not forced.

ANAL TOYS

The anus has many nerve endings, and many men and women find anal stimulation as exciting as genital stimulation. There is also a diverse range of sex toys for this area that we can use if we want to innovate our sexual practices. For safety reasons, every anal toy must have a smooth surface with no seams, and a wider base to avoid total insertion into the interior of the rectum, which causes major problems. Some smaller toys are designed so you can leave them inside and thus have free hands to continue with intercourse or caressing other parts of your partner's body.

Use objects with a small diameter to start with and, as you begin feeling comfortable, increase the size. There are inflatable vibrators that are a good resource because their size can be changed and cause great pleasure when they inflate via a knob on the exterior. In order to deflate them you just have to open the valve and let the air out.